Cracking the Menopause

To our mothers who made us think, to our sisters and friends who made us talk, and to our daughters who made us want to change their world.

Cracking the Menopause

While keeping yourself together

Mariella Frostrup
Alice Smellie

bluebird
books for life

First published 2021 by Bluebird
an imprint of Pan Macmillan
The Smithson, 6 Briset Street, London EC1M 5NR
EU representative: Macmillan Publishers Ireland Ltd,
1st Floor, The Liffey Trust Centre, 117–126 Sheriff Street Upper,
Dublin 1, D01 YC43
Associated companies throughout the world
www.panmacmillan.com

HB ISBN 978-1-5290-5903-8
TPB ISBN 978-1-5290-5904-5

1 3 5 7 9 8 6 4 2

A CIP catalogue record for this book is available from the British Library.

Typeset in Kepler Std by Palimpsest Book Production Ltd, Falkirk, Stirlingshire
Printed and bound by CPI Group (UK) Ltd, Croydon, CR0 4YY

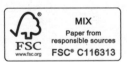

The information provided in this book is not an alternative to medical advice
from your doctor or other professional healthcare provider. You should not
delay in seeking medical advice, disregard medical advice or discontinue any
medical treatment because of the information provided in this book.

Visit **www.panmacmillan.com** to read more about all our books
and to buy them. You will also find features, author interviews and
news of any author events, and you can sign up for e-newsletters
so that you're always first to hear about our new releases.

Contents

Preface

For me, menopause felt like being sucked into a black hole. I had no bearings and changing course was not an option. Having left school in my mid-teens, I initially assumed that I'd simply missed, or skipped, the relevant biology class. But that lesson had never taken place. Even for those who lingered in the education system, the end result would be the same. Most of us have moved through our lives ignorant of what menopause is and what it will mean, and we remain blissfully oblivious until we're bowled over by symptoms and forced to embark on a crash course.

That was certainly my experience. At what seemed like the reasonably young age of fifty-one, I reached the full stop that every woman is told to dread. Through the centuries, menopause has been the hormonal catastrophe that stalks every woman's life. It's mostly unmentionable and ignored until the day your monthly cycle ends, and with it your fertility and supposedly much more besides. It was shocking to discover that although I felt I was simply beginning a sixth decade of life, the place at which I'd arrived was perceived as a living death. How could I have been ignorant for so long about this elephant's graveyard for my sex, where we all wind up once we've served our useful time?

Presenting menopause as a cosmic-scale gravity chasm may be taking a slight liberty, but that's what it still represents for many of us. I felt the oppressive proximity of an inevitable future of dried-up sexual organs, hot flushes, lack of desirability, general shrivelling, and ultimately loss of brain power and death. Psychologists warn against fight-or-flight mode, yet I found myself trapped in an unwinnable conflict with my own hormones.

In a hilarious sketch 'Last F**kable Day', the comedian Amy

Schumer brutally but sharply illustrates how ageing instantly renders us menopausal women undesirable to men overnight.[1] With symptoms like insomnia and anxiety taking their toll, desirability certainly wasn't in my top ten of worries, but 'Brazen Husky', as the *Daily Mail* once summed up my charms,[2] was certainly not what the world was seeing now! Flailing around for helpful information merely confirmed that the end of life as I'd previously known it was beckoning.

After a lifetime spent in frank discussion about every aspect of women's lives, the near-total silence from women surrounding this mysterious moment seemed even more ominous. When I was sixteen and living in Catholic Ireland, my mother helped me acquire the pill. She and I had talked about sex and death, divorce and bad periods, we'd battled her cervical cancer together and discussed the meaning of life when she was diagnosed with dementia, but we'd never, ever, ever talked about the menopause.

My only recollection of her mentioning this transitory period of her life was a fleeting comment in my late twenties about a hormone patch she had used. This, she said, made her feel like an un-milked dairy cow – bloated and uncomfortable – a sliver of information that served to instil further foreboding. Nothing to look forward to there . . . Aside from that, even in our most vocal of households, it was the closest we ever got to discussing this compulsory progression in every woman's biological journey.

Although I think of it as a staging post rather than a final destination, our culture still says otherwise. Puberty and pregnancy are seen as positive progressions, but menopause is when forward momentum halts and, like Shakespeare's 'golden lads and girls', we begin to 'come to dust.'[3] Though, notably, men mature, while us dusty women wither and shrivel.

In some ways, it's understandable that menopause should be deemed such a traumatic rite of passage. Our fertility is so deeply embedded in our psyches that, for many women, it feels like our entire *raison d'être*. Suffering setbacks in pursuit of procreation or choosing to eschew it altogether can ultimately feel like a bereavement or a failure, as many women who've struggled with infertility, not met the right partner, or decided not to have children may have found. We've been told for millennia that our only point is to procreate, and we're made to feel it leaves a big gap on our CV if we won't, haven't, or can't. As a result, menopause has culturally come to render women redundant, unlike any middle-aged man in the prime of his life.

With women's issues of health, wealth, rights and happiness on the menu as never before, it's high time we dragged this third stage of our biological cycle out of the depths of Pandora's Box. Despite Homo sapiens spending more than 200,000 years on this planet,[4] menopause appears to have been less explored than the Mariana Trench:[5] misdiagnosed, misappropriated and misunderstood in a narrative composed almost entirely by men. Half the world's population is affected, but it remains one of the most toxic words in our lexicon, signalling the end of a woman's worth and value, the loss of libido, the shrivelling up of organs and the final fast track to decline and death. With our increasing lifespans – we're often living almost as long again after our final period passes – for the majority of us, menopause occurs midway through our lives, leaving us with a generous and exciting second phase of existence.

All of which suggests that now, in the twenty-first century, with most women's lives unrecognizable from what they were even a century ago, it's time to change the negative and end-of-days dynamic.

Introduction

I know I speak for many women when I say that if menopause were a place you could elect to visit, it wouldn't be popular. Most of us arrive in a state of surprise and then trepidation. Having thought for years that I was a reasonably well-informed woman of the world, menopause knocked that assumption firmly aside. The lack of clear direction is quite staggering. What we need is straightforward navigation. But I, like so many of us, found myself stumbling solo through a maze of misinformation and confusion, without so much as a compass to show me the way.

I've spoken a great deal about opening the conversation, and I still believe that we need to talk more openly. Menopause was a chat I'd never had; not with my mother, my friends or even my GP. I knew the word, and had a vague start date in mind, around my fiftieth birthday. Other than that, my scant knowledge could have been jotted on one of my mother's short-lived HRT patches.

So, when I started to notice symptoms at the age of forty-nine, I had no idea what was happening. For two years I hardly slept a wink, raged at my husband and kids, and was swamped by levels of anxiety that were as debilitating as they were irrational. I don't think I've ever felt so alone. On the rare occasions when I mentioned my concerns to girlfriends ('I slept four hours last night, is this normal?'), they all seemed to have more questions than answers, just like me.

Sadly, this is the unfortunate experience for millions of women. We all know loosely what 'menopause' means but are ignorant of specifics – most importantly that symptoms might start years before the event itself, during what's known as the perimenopause. In a UK survey[1] of one thousand women, seventy per cent of participants said they'd experienced perimenopausal symptoms in their thirties and forties, yet ninety per cent of these failed to rapidly recognize the link to their fluctuating hormones – taking on average fourteen months to join the dots.

What a strange anomaly this is. We're not thirteen-year-old girls bemused by our changing bodies. We are intelligent professionals who manage our finances, do our own washing and know how to put air into car tyres (though some of us are a bit rusty . . . brain fog?). But most of us are as perplexed as any teen in a training bra when it comes to details about this major date in our fertility calendar.

Eventually, aged fifty-one, a mere shadow of my former self, I went to see Sara Matthews, my gynaecologist. I've raved in the past about her Jessica Rabbit-like elegance and tumbling Titian locks. But more important than her glamour – and, actually, I yearned for glamour as I was feeling so utterly drab – was the feeling of coming home, as I sat down in her office and started to describe how I felt. Not only did she hear me, but she immediately identified the problem. I was, without question, perimenopausal.

Once I realized that I was experiencing the menopause, I felt as though I'd stumbled on the world's best-kept secret. What became rapidly evident was that, as with 'natural birth', managing the symp-toms of menopause by gritting your teeth and getting on with it (and definitely not discussing it in public) seemed to have become the litmus test for admirable stoic femininity. So I started to ask questions.

If menopause was barely mentioned among women, it was posi-tively banned in the company of men. The only acceptable references were lewd comments in yawnsome stand-up comedian monologues and tepid sitcoms, where menopause and mother-in-law jokes have provided easy targets since time immemorial. 'Why is menopause called menopause? Because mad cow disease was taken' is a prime example. Laugh? I think not. Making women feel marginalized and humiliated is no longer palatable.

It seemed that we were fifty per cent of the population of the whole world, but were deemed an 'invisible minority'. Could things really be this cataclysmic? In 2018, I set out to find answers, making a BBC1 documentary called *The Truth About the Menopause*. We barely scratched the surface of this huge topic, as television tends to do, but I was overwhelmed with the tsunami of gratitude – and viewing figures to match.

Women scurried up to me in bars, restaurants, in the workplace, on the Tube, in public toilets, in the cinema and in the queue at the chemist, whispering their secrets and their gratitude as though in the confession box.

To my amusement, at a film party in London, the handsome actor Michael Fassbender was pushed unceremoniously aside by a woman in her thirties, who wanted to enthuse about my use of the M-word, leaving me to explain to Michael why the menopause matters so much! I wonder if he's recovered.

Most of the time I felt utterly astonished at having done so little to provoke such a great response. Rather than feeling pride in my supposedly pioneering exposé, I felt even angrier that this liminal phase in our lives, something so mundane and inevitable, should be the wellspring of so much shame, anxiety, ignorance and fear. Once the conversation was started, and we were talking, it appeared that all women had something to say.

In chapter one, we'll take a whirlwind tour through the mostly pitiful, ignorant and certainly highly biased 'information' that's swirled around us over the last few thousand years. Chapter two onwards will take you through all things menopause in the modern age, with contributions from women with many different experiences. It's time to drag menopause and all the surrounding symptoms and experiences out into the sunlight. Only by talking, by airing and sharing, listening and learning will we progress from the position of ignorance we've been relegated to for so long.

Now I've talked, I very firmly believe it's time to act.

CHAPTER ONE

Myth and Menopause

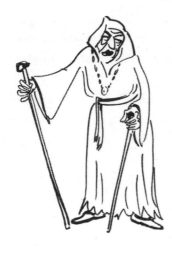

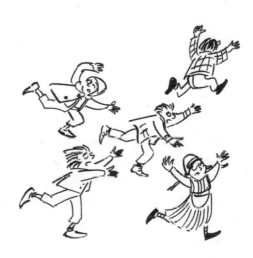

*'Poisonous and dangerous, with the ability
to kill children just by looking at them.'*

Pointless and poisonous: the first millennia

Where do you start, with centuries of ignorant assumption and ludicrous diagnosis to condense into a few historical snapshots? Happily, we don't have to plunge back into the primordial swamps, as there isn't much reference to older women's bodies until the seventeenth century. Menopause is very much a medical afterthought, from classical times onwards. Being unique to women, it was obviously unimportant and uninteresting unless it impacted on the lives of the ruling classes, who were, almost to a man, men. I say this with heavy sarcasm, which is laced with unassailable truth.

Looking back through the arch of history, you certainly come to the conclusion that menopause needs a spin doctor. In 1969, the American doctor David Reuben, in his bestseller *Everything You Always Wanted to Know About Sex*,[1] offers a rare snippet of 'positivity' by informing us that, 'As oestrogen is shut off a woman becomes as close as she can to being a man,' (that's the good news), with the caveat that, 'Having outlived their ovaries, they may have outlived their usefulness as human beings'. Less good. And Reuben is allegedly on our side. But this is the tone that is common throughout the ages. There's a 'Whoops, it's all over love' subtext to almost every written word or comment made about the end of female fertility, whether it be medical or literary.

Peering back to the first dim documentation certainly compounds the sense of looming disaster. If periods were called the 'curse', then what followed was nothing short of a death sentence!

Let's start with ancient times: those wonderful Greek and Roman men who were eternally immortalized in marble and are still studied by classics students. It's unlikely you'll be able to conjure up any female names.

Unsurprisingly, the menopause wasn't prominent in their medical research or philosophical theories. Greek philosopher and revered thinker Aristotle managed one nearly accurate bit of detail around 300 BC, saying the average age at which fertility ceased was around forty, but it definitely happened by fifty.[2] In fact, fifty-one is the average age at which we have our final period. In terms of consistency, the time of menopause appears to be one of the most stable incidences in human biology.

There was certainly no interest expressed about perimenopause, the years preceding the menopause itself, when hormones start to go up and down like an opinion poll about the top ten hottest Greek gods.

I'd be tempted to scrutinize Aristotle's pioneering philosophies with a stern eye if they are anything like as flawed as his description of women's bodies. According to him, women contain too much blood due to our coldness, general ineptitude, and less active lifestyle. Periods are the process of getting rid of the excess blood, whereas men – of course – are constructed with perfect balance and just the right amount of heat and blood (which they make into semen).[3] This idea of menstruation as a cleansing process of some sort endures for almost another two thousand years. (Incidentally, Aristotle thought of a woman as a 'mutilated male'.)

> I'd be tempted to scrutinize Aristotle's pioneering philosophies with a stern eye if they are anything like as flawed as his description of women's bodies. According to him, women contain too much blood due to our coldness, general lack of ability, and less active lifestyle.

David Reuben was toward the end of a long line of 'experts' to offer the opinion that, as women go beyond menopause and their periods stop, they become more masculine, though, as he says, 'Not really a man, but no longer a functional woman'. In some societies, including Ancient Greece, there were (and still are) freedoms given to post-menopausal women – as a reward, one presumes, for getting so close to the idealized marvellousness of men.

As we move on through the centuries, interest in the menopause remains pretty static, a disinterested medical shrug. A sixth-century physician, Aetius, suggested that the 'very fat cease early'[4] (untrue, as it happens), and the 'first' female gynaecologist, Trotula of Salerno, was a voice of reason around the eleventh century in Italy. It's said that she wrote a major work on women's medicine in medieval Europe, *On the Diseases of Women*. Or did she? Did she exist? Was she in fact a man? Historians simply cannot agree on this point.[5] I am pretty sure that, had she been a man, there'd be clear documentation and a large medical school in his name, with a big statue outside. The Father of Gynaecology, he'd be called. Instead, there's an ongoing debate: 'We're unsure. Was Trotula a woman or a pseudonym?'

Then there's Saint Hildegard of Bingen in twelfth-century Germany, who was staggeringly pioneering. Her observation, 'the menses cease in woman from the fiftieth year and sometimes in certain ones from the sixtieth when the uterus begins to be enfolded and to contract so they are no longer able to conceive,'[6] may not be entirely accurate, but is not that far removed from our level of understanding today. Hildegard, who wrote classical music that is still played today and founded two abbeys, very much flew the flag for post-menopausal success. Aged sixty, she went on four preaching tours, in spite of women having been forbidden to do so. And at least she was a member of the female sex, with hands-on experience, rather than one of the numerous mumbling men who felt qualified to offer their unqualified opinions on all matters female over the centuries.

Moving on up through our bloody – literally – history, in the Middle Ages our inability to get rid of what was considered toxic blood meant that menopausal women were seen as bubbling cauldrons of poisons. We didn't have the strength to expel them, and suffered terribly, till we dropped dead from one of the many venoms we harboured.

The thirteenth-century German philosopher and scientist, Albertus Magnus, whose day job was 'German Catholic Dominican Bishop', wrote a dark tome called *De Secretis Mulierum* (*Women's Secrets*). This cheery book was filled with insights such as, 'The retention of menses engenders many evil humours'.[7]

Magnus – and I think it's fair to suggest that he wasn't exactly a jolly family man – also believed that older women were poisonous and dangerous, with the ability to kill children just by looking at them. Sometimes, when a teen is being particularly infuriating, and begging to stay on at a party, for example, it would be a useful threat. 'Midnight, or I come in and LOOK at you.' What a typical menopausal reference though. The moment it's remotely interesting to medics, academics and men – same thing – it's evident that it's judged to be a scourge rather than a liberation. Typically, his flagrant inaccuracies didn't stand in the way of his career success; Magnus was later canonized as Saint Albert the Great, patron saint of the natural sciences.[8]

The sixteenth-century Italian doctor Giovanni Marinello, in *Le medicine partenenti alle infermità delle donne*, which roughly translates as 'Medicine for Women's Problems' (1563), gives a less witchy, more medical, but nonetheless utterly dismal description of any woman whose periods have halted.

> Those women [ladies, that's you] . . . are always infirm and most of all in those parts of the body which are connected to and have some kind of correspondence with the uterus . . . thus as soon as the periods stop, pains arise, apostemata, eye disorders, weak sight, vomiting, fever; and they desire the male more than ever.[9]

Ah, yes. You'll notice the mention of us desiring men. Another repulsive trait of menopausal women through the ages is our desperation for sex. During our fecund (fuckable) days, such interest in the male of the species might possibly be something to celebrate, but not when it's a menopausal hag doing the lusting.

Marinello continues for quite some time in the same vein:

> The disorderly uterus rises or descends all the time or commits other actions difficult to endure. From this soon a tightness of the chest arises, faintings of the heart, breathlessness, hiccups, and other troublesome accidents, from which the woman sometimes dies. Also spitting of blood, haemorrhoids, and, especially in maidens, copious nose bleeding come from it, and endless other ills, which we think too many to relate.

Even for his time, Marinello displays a penchant for exaggeration. The symptoms of menopause are diverse and the effects of declining hormones known to be extensive, but even without a medical degree I know for a fact that 'spitting of blood' doesn't appear on any list of symptoms.

Despite having been accomplished healers throughout history, particularly in the areas of periods and childbirth, often women weren't officially welcomed as medical experts, were barred from universities and – if born in the wrong century – likely to be accused of witchcraft.[10] Many an innocent with a good knowledge of herbal remedies spent time on a ducking stool, or worse. In her pioneering book, *Hot Flushes, Cold Science*, Louise Foxcroft explains that eighty per cent of those put to death for witchcraft were female, and most were older women. 'Post-menopausal women were particularly vulnerable as they no longer served the purpose of procreation. If widowed, they neither fulfilled the role of wife, nor were they protected by a husband from malicious accusations, and women who inherited property violated the common expectations that wealth should pass down the male line.'[11]

The idea that ageing equalled a pact with the Devil was challenged by the English MP Reginald Scot. In *The Discovery of Witchcraft* (1584), he said that post-menopausal women were particularly at risk of being accused of the crime 'upon the stopping of their monthly melancholic flux or issue of blood', as this made them 'falsely suppose' that they could 'hurt and enfeeble men's bodies'. In today's language, that probably means that they had their own opinions.

Scot – bless the man – said that witchcraft didn't exist and that the women under suspicion were just old and poor.[12] Nonetheless, around 200,000 women in Western Europe were tortured or executed in the three hundred years up to 1750.

To drag a lone positive from this seething quagmire of negativity, the concept of our blood was seen as disgusting, but, by the late eighteenth century, the idea of it being actively venomous was over. Now, menopause was medicalized as a terrible illness to be feared and treated.[13] Things were – I'm sure you'll agree – progressing.

Irrational and sex crazed: the next stage

Welcome to the nineteenth century. It's probably thirty million years since we crawled from the seas, and a few million years since humans appeared,[14] yet we're still no closer to understanding women's later biological life. Crucially, though, this was the age during which menopause was formally identified. Before you start calling hallelujah for wider understanding, this was also a time during which you were likely to be given a spell in the lunatic asylum for yelling at your husband. Thankfully, women aren't still subject to such restraints – or I'd be facing my golden years sporting a straitjacket and rocking backwards and forwards in a padded cell.

It was a French doctor who coined the word 'menopause'. Charles Pierre Louis de Gardanne first came up with it in 1821 in his must-read book, *De la ménopause, ou de l'âge critique des femmes* (*Menopause: The Critical Age of Women*). By 1824, it was in a French medical dictionary.[15]

The word itself comes from the Greek; *menos* actually means month and *pausis* means pause or cease.[16] Put like that, of course it doesn't sound quite so dramatic. Incidentally, the French may have come up with that fairly bland term, but they also conceived '*l'enfer des femmes*' – 'the hell of women' – and described menopausal women as '*des reines dethrones*' – 'dethroned queens'.[17]

Although the Industrial Revolution, which was tootling along at the same time, was transforming working lives, for women it was the same old story. The Victorians, in the age of machines and at the height of an era of advancement and progress (although a massive thumbs down to the Empire and all that entailed), postulated that women's minds are feeble and weak, and we're susceptible to madness, because of our malfunctioning (for which read 'penis free') bodies.

Menopause was finally discussed, which you'd think a positive, and the perimenopause – the years leading up to the final point – was now generally identified as the 'climacteric'.

Medics were recommending pills and potions for the many symptoms (the monetizing of the menopause had very much begun!), but the fact that medicine understood more about our physiology didn't necessarily do us any favours. 'Ovulation fixes women's place in the animal economy,' said one fun doctor in 1880.[18]

By the middle of the nineteenth century, doctors pretty much linked anything menstrual, ovary or womb-themed with madness and hysteria, especially if you were drawing near to the end of your cycles. At no time were women more likely to become unstable, the men said grimly, than around this time. As you lost your one useful purpose, you also lost your marbles and even your health. Such a typical double whammy; as a woman, you were damned if you were having periods, but even more so if they were stopping. Obviously, I acknowledge mood swings, but these are not to be dismissed as end-of-life flailings.

'Insanity frequently occurs at the change of constitution,' agreed the obstetrician and writer W. Tyler Smith in his 1849 article, *The Climacteric Disease in Women; A Paroxysmal Affection Occurring at the Decline of the Catamenia* (I think the clue is in the title). 'I have no doubt that it is often owing to the climacteric paroxysms. Each paroxysm is a distinct shock to the brain, leaving behind it peevishness, irritability of temper and eccentricity.'[19]

One 1830s physician was adamant that menopause was a clear prelude to depression and death: 'There is a predisposition to many diseases, and these are often of a melancholy character,' he stated.[20] Again, a potentially amusing misunderstanding of women's bodies that fails to raise a laugh, because we are still more likely to be prescribed antidepressants than have menopause properly diagnosed.

As well as being insane and ill, once menopause had us in its grip, we were ugly. Women, when they became incapable of conceiving, were now seen to become masculine and repulsive. In 1882, the English doctor Edward Tilt, who wrote the first English book dealing with 'climacteric disorders' in 1857, said that you could spot a menopausal woman a mile off. 'The complexion is pale or sallow, or there may be a drowsy look, or the dull, stupid astonishment of one seeking to rouse herself to answer a question.'[21] There's also a tendency to sprout hair on the upper lip and chin (the latter a fair point, especially if you add testosterone to your HRT cocktail – of which more later!).

Sadly, as we became more repulsive, physicians of the time again noted that we were also driven mad with desperate and strange desires. In 1870, the psychiatrist Henry Maudsley described menopausal libido as 'A disease by which the most chaste and modest woman is transformed into a raging fury of lust.'[22] Although a small proportion of women find their libido off the scale in the last throes of fertility, I'd say his description still sounds like male optimism.

Staying calm and domesticated was good for our health, as Elaine Showalter points out in her book, *The Female Malady* (although society continues to seem hell-bent on making that a challenge).[23] It was felt that too much education for women, or trying to emulate the strength and ambition of men, could precipitate mental breakdown. Incidentally, the word 'hysteria' comes from the Greek for the womb – naturally.

> In 1870, the psychiatrist Henry Maudsley described menopausal libido as 'A disease by which the most chaste and modest woman is transformed into a raging fury of lust.'

'Education, attempts at birth control or abortion, undue sexual indulgence, a too-fashionable lifestyle, failure to devote herself fully to the needs of husband and children – even the advocacy of suffrage – all might guarantee a disease-ridden menopause,' says Carroll Smith-Rosenburg of nineteenth-century attitudes in 'Puberty to Menopause: The Cycle of Femininity in Nineteenth-Century America' (1973).[24] It's all our fault, ladies! Perhaps the best title for a turn of the century book about the subject might have been, 'Cry Votes For Women and Die Young' . . .

Cure or kill

Because it was seen as a disease, menopause therefore needed to be cured. Some of the therapies sounded staggeringly foul – and far more dangerous and disconcerting than any hot flush or sleepless night. At no time were 'cures' more thoroughly and horrifically investigated than in the late nineteenth century, when the menopause was being explored as a medical condition. I use the term 'investigated' advisedly. I think the kindest word for the science explored is 'experimental'.

W. Tyler Smith's patronizing tone is reflective of the era. 'Heavy and prolonged sleep, particularly in the morning, exerts a marked influence in increasing the severity and frequency of the paroxysms,' he says firmly.[25] A paroxysm is defined as 'a sudden attack or outburst of a particular emotion or activity', which could, I suppose, be anything from a snapped 'Bugger off!' to kicking your physician in the shins.

As is so often the case with the 'speculative fiction' about menopause, that was clearly written by a man with no idea that you can go to bed at nine p.m., sweat your way through most of the night and wind up having had only three hours of actual rest. What menopausal woman wouldn't welcome a lie in, sleep deprivation being one of a myriad of symptoms. But you can't help wondering if he simply had an eye on all the jobs that wouldn't get done with women spending their days just lying in bed feeling sorry for themselves or lusting after the opposite sex, despite their arid repulsiveness!

For those of you who, like me, can't get enough of his 'insights', there's more: 'All violent mental emotion should be carefully avoided,' and, 'Stimulating diet and stimulating drinks should be used only with the utmost caution'. He's just one small step away from advising that, post-fifty, we be put down.

Tyler Smith also liked to get his hands dirty, and he particularly delights in describing with eye-watering and vampiric glee the bene-fits of bloodletting from the womb. Without going into too much detail, suffice it to say that it involves applying three or four leeches to the cervical area. Further joyful solutions included ice in the vagina and cold-water injections into the rectum.

From a twenty-first-century female point of view, the very thought of most of these 'cures' would be enough for me to say quite firmly that I was just fine, free of all my feminine wiles (or should that be viles?), and promise to live out my remaining years very quietly, under the radar, so as not to disturb men any further with my offensive presence. Perhaps this is one reason why we've got to the twenty-first century without clear illumination and focus on menopause. It's as good an explanation as any other for the silence surrounding this most guaranteed of female evolutionary biological processes.

Incidentally, as is so often the case, any patient's experience of vaginal leeching (good or bad) remains unrecorded. I couldn't find any 'tried and tested' reviews available from those subjected to Tyler Smith's treatments, but I suspect he would have fared pretty poorly on Instagram likes.

He wasn't the only medic pioneering seemingly sadistic, or just plain silly treatments. Edward Tilt also recommended some quite eye-watering solutions for our failing bodies. 'Camphor . . . seems to correct the toxic influence which the reproductive system has on the brain of some women.' Going one step (or staircase) further, he says that, 'In some cases of perverted cerebral innervation, the inhalation of chloroform, or of a mixture of chloroform and ether, may be use-fully carried to the verge of unconsciousness.' And who wouldn't like a vaginal or rectal suppository of opiates . . . Tilt also talks lightly of the application of leeches to the anus or ears. Or six to eight – count 'em – leeches on the perineum.[26]

American surgeon Andrew Currier advocated simple problem-solving in the 1890s by whipping out the ovaries and causing artificial menopause.[27] There were plenty of such unnecessary-sounding operations performed, with an overwhelming air of 'might as well give it a go' about the whole thing and a high degree of trial and error, but scant regard for expert knowledge. Would such experimentation have been similarly indulged if it was killing off men, I wonder?

Although most of these investigations sound like the work of focused psychopaths, there was some method in the apparent madness of these doctors. Occasionally, they'd pioneer a treatment which would result in genuine breakthrough. In the early 1890s, for example, a French scientist injected a menopausal patient with ovarian extract to cure her 'madness', and three years later, in 1896, a German physician used desiccated ovaries as a 'cure'.[28]

These rudimentary experiments represented a step forward in the search for solutions. HRT, or Hormone Replacement Therapy, today is of course made from substances that mimic female hormones.

As for information from women themselves, aside from rare female perspectives such as Trotula (who might have been a man) and Hildegard, there are few clues as to our thoughts on this singularly female experience.

We see occasional shafts of light, suggesting that women themselves were relieved to be free of periods and pregnancies, that older women might be useful within the family and at work, and that, once the menopause was over, we might enjoy a peaceful old age. Never equal to men, naturally, but at least not entirely redundant. When your chances of dying in childbirth were so high, dicing with death on a biannual basis must have made menopause a blessed relief for many of the sorority.

Bottoms up! What were they 'thinking'?

In the early twentieth century, the emergence of psychoanalysis did women no favours. Sigmund Freud is perhaps most famous for his 1933 penis-envy theory, but he also said, 'It's a well-known fact . . .

that after women have lost their genital function their character often undergoes a peculiar alteration'.[29]

Sadly, this personality change didn't mean we could object to men making unsubstantiated statements about our physiology. Freud further added, as though we hadn't endured enough, that we 'become quarrelsome and obstinate, petty and stingy, show typical and anal-erotic features which they did not show before.'[30] He must have been such a blast at dinner parties; I know I would have called up in advance and begged to be seated next to him.

In fairness, it's not only men who have opined negatively about our journey into the next phase of womanhood. A student of Freud's, the psychiatrist Helene Deutsch, referred to the menopause as – variously – 'partial death', the 'natural end as servant of the species' and a period of 'psychological distress'.[31] She's actually right about the latter, but that's mainly down to the inexhaustible supply of gloomy mythology to which she seems to have enthusiastically contributed. Again, she must have made any book-club evening with the girls and a bottle of wine a light-hearted romp.

Our lack of ability to think coherently at this time of life meant that menopause could even be used in court. A paper published in 1999 covered this quite extraordinary subject. 'Because of the menopause, m'lud,' was used from 1900 to the 1980s in the United States, and the 'menopause defence' was actually taken seriously in some cases of divorce and serious injury. The first documented reference to menopause in a reported legal decision was in Texas in 1900, where a gas company unsuccessfully alleged that injuries sustained by a woman who fell into an uncovered trench were due to her menstrual problems rather than the fall.[32]

Famous feminist Simone de Beauvoir was also pretty mournful about menopause (and ageing generally), which she calls 'the dangerous age'. Writing in *The Second Sex* (1949), she pointed out that, 'While the male grows older continuously, the woman is brusquely stripped of her femininity . . . Well before the definitive mutilation, woman is haunted by the fear of growing old.' Happily, once through the portal and on the other side, she's a mite less pessimistic. 'It has been far less sombre,' she pondered, 'than I had foreseen.'

Less helpfully, she also focuses on the theme of us returning to girlishness, saying of the menopausal woman: 'In a pathetic effort, she tries to stop time . . . She ostentatiously brings up her memories of girlhood; instead of speaking, she chirps, she claps her hands, she bursts out laughing.'[33]

This sort of return to adolescence is referenced throughout nineteenth-century writing as well, and is just as patronizing and insulting as any 'hysteric' label.

Staying pretty in the sixties

And then in the mid-twentieth century we struck gold. It's over to the States and HRT for all. The time had come to hold onto your bonnets and stay pretty, little ladies! Menopause was a deficiency disease, but no worries, as long as you take the drugs. In the swinging Sixties, HRT was all the rage, and in 1966 the American gynaecologist Robert A. Wilson, MD, who published a book called *Feminine Forever*, told us why.[34] His unequivocal viewpoint . . . that ladies needed to remain young and fun, or they'd lose their husbands, and quite right too.

Wilson, no great shakes in the looks department himself, since we're chucking insults around, charmlessly refers to the menopausal state as 'living decay', with some quite staggering claims. The menopause is apparently 'curable' and also 'completely preventable'; and why wouldn't you want to stop it in its tracks, as 'the unpalatable truth must be faced that all post-menopausal women are castrates'. That's right. We're men without testicles. Not women.

Interestingly, Wilson references his own experience, which included 'the tragic decline of my gentle, almost angelic, mother . . . I was appalled at the transformation of that vital, wonderful woman who had been the dynamic focal point of our family into a pain-racked, petulant invalid.'

Wilson's book is still famous, and is always referenced in histories of the menopause, although he's not viewed as the helpful prophet I suspect he felt himself to be. Helpful to whom, one has to ask; certainly not the fifty per cent of the population being misinformed and mistreated as a result of continuing levels of ignorance. I think it's useful if you want to see how much worse attitudes to women were last century, but otherwise, definitely not. There are days when I feel as though I exist in a state of living decay, but it's not sex specific, Mr Wilson. Looking at the men around me is a welcome reminder that ageing happens to us all.

Most significantly, Wilson calls the menopause a 'tragedy'. Poor us. 'A woman's awareness of her femininity completely suffuses her character and . . . the tragedy of menopause often destroys her character as well as her health.'

On the bright side, he appears to be genuinely promoting education about the subject, and trying to ease symptoms. However, describing menopause as a 'mutilation of the whole body' is neither helpful nor illuminating. This sort of negative wording just adds Wilson to the long line of male observers of this specifically female phase who have no real idea what they are talking about. May I also add that Wilson had a financial interest in HRT? Persuading all women to embrace it to prevent this state of mutilation and save our husbands from our ill humour will presumably have added a few noughts to his bank account.

In the 1970s, in the second wave of feminism, there was a backlash, when us pushy women insisted that we too had a voice. We pointed out, with some vehemence, that menopause was just part of the natural process of ageing and it should stop being treated like an inevitable illness. 'Even today the literature . . . defines menopause as a deficiency disease . . . It certainly echoes once more the male prejudice against menopausal and post-menopausal women,' said a 1977 article.

Women, on the other hand, argued that it could be rather marvellous. 'Because menopause freed women from the risk of pregnancy, it was viewed as a sexually liberating event,' said writer Frances McCrea in 1983.[35] And yet, 'The ageing woman has a particularly vulnerable status in our society . . . To blame all the problems that ageing women experience on menopause is a classic case of blaming the victim.'

Has much really changed? The fact is that, until very recently, women have experienced menopause and men have had opinions about it. For hundreds of years it has been documented and treated by those who haven't had so much as a twinge of period pain, never mind experienced monthly bleeding, pregnancy and childbirth.

That's not to say that *every* observation made down the centuries has been incorrect, but many of them are. In direct contrast to the decline in our oestrogen levels, the tsunami of inaccurate and negative mythology has continued to rise. If I have an agenda, it's to turn back the tide of misrepresentation which is overwhelming my own sex in unnecessary fear and apprehension, as well as totally misleading the rest of the population about a natural, entirely survivable and potentially liberating phase of our lives. A friend's husband has described childbirth as 'smarting a bit'. This level of ignorance sums up the problem with letting men's observations define women's menopause.

Today, over three thousand years on from the Pharoah Rameses II correctly pointing out that there was no point in trying to help a sixty-year-old woman conceive, and following four waves of feminism,[36] one of the few absolutes for most women, apart from death, is that we will experience the menopause. Yet it remains a dirty word, whispered in dark corners, avoided in conversation and still certainly not on the menu in civilized company. How are we ever to understand what's happening to our bodies when the outcome of centuries of propaganda is that we're often too ashamed to admit to ourselves that change is occurring?

> A friend's husband has described childbirth as 'smarting a bit'. This level of ignorance sums up the problem with letting men's observations define women's menopause.

Phyllis Kernoff Mansfield, Professor Emeritus of Women's Studies at Penn State University, who has authored many studies about menopausal attitudes,[37] asked the question, in 1998: 'Why do women continue to feel they don't know anything about menopause? Because every woman's menopause is unique and no study has validated that uniqueness,' thereby summing up the biggest single issue with how we treat menopause today.

In the next chapter, we'll talk about what the word actually means, rather than what it's come to mean, but, in short, the definition of 'menopause' is the twelve-month anniversary of your last period. As a way to describe the potential ten years of biological turbulence preceding that auspicious date, and the further fine-tuning that carries on afterwards, it's misleading and even redundant.

Using menopause as a catch-all term for every ailment a woman might experience from her mid-forties onwards is a classic example of the herd assumptions that continue to be applied to our sex. This natural biological progression, a waypoint, that will affect each and every one of us in entirely different ways, is scooped up, mislabelled, under-examined and misdiagnosed. Culturally and medically, it's regarded as an ending, rather than a new beginning. It's high time we rallied together and refused to allow our functioning lives to be so unfairly foreshortened.

Language speaks volumes, and the term 'menopause' still carries a lot of dead weight. The end of our periods is the signal that we've been through a biological reboot, yet too often treatment only comes at the end of that passage. Most of us will need some support for the sake of ourselves, our families and our careers. So why are we still so afraid to ask for it?

It's high time we renovated and elevated this life change. Despite the centuries of speculation and propaganda, we are not overheating or inherently cold, we are not hysterics or boiling vats of toxic poisons, we are not dried up or washed up, we are simply menopausal. Far from shutting down, having made that progression, we can open up to feeling freer, braver and more liberated than ever before. Understanding what's happening and ensuring that our health, both mental and physical, becomes a priority is what will make it a story with a happy ending. That's what this book is dedicated to achieving.

Did you know medicine is for men?

Medicine is, and always has been, sexist, being completely biased towards the male form. The spare-rib theory has informed medical attitudes since the dawn of time, and it's only now, in the twenty-first century, that the health system is waking up to the physiological differences between males and females. It's an outrage that women might be diagnosed with anxiety rather than a heart attack because our symptoms don't resemble those of men, and we are therefore 'atypical'. If medicine is unable to acknowledge that women's bodies are very different to those of men, what hope of being taken seriously when we're going through a hormonal catastrophe, specific to the female of the species, and one that affects us as much emotionally as it does physically?

Irrational, angry, hysterical, depressed and even senile are just some of the words I've seen applied to women who were simply trying to navigate physiological turbulence during their body's metamorphosis. From our cradles to our graves, there currently exists a disastrous level of ignorance about female biological make-up, and menopause specifically.

Our flawed hormones

MEDICAL FEMINIST, NHS GP DR SARAH HILLMAN:

On the day I did my TEDx Talk about Medical Feminism, in 2019, there were fifteen other talks, many of them about controversial topics. All were fascinating and valid experiences which deserved insight and understanding. But when the talks were made public on YouTube, while the other talks received almost exclusively positive comments, mine were initially very negative: 'Nothing worse than a female doctor who can't relate to a massively muscular athletic male,' said one. 'How'd she graduate medical school and not know there's chemotherapy to cure feminism?' snarked another.

There is appalling gender discrepancy throughout the medical profession, which was founded by men and focused on men, and has endured for thousands of years. There are fewer female senior doctors and professors, and there is a significant gender pay gap. Change in or add the word 'ethnicity', and you compound the problem.

Clinical studies into medicines are historically based on the seventy-kilogram male, in part because of the inconvenient nature of women's fluctuating hormones. This even applies to animal models; obviously female mice have ovaries too. Rather than taking female organs into account, they've been dismissed, and it is perhaps the reason I see women suffering side effects to quite standard drugs, until we reduce or adjust the dose.

Gender bias also plays a role when it comes to those who conduct research, as well as those who participate in a study. In Canada, the Institute of Health Research conducted an experiment. They looked at the research grant applications and found that, when reviewers of the proposals assessed the science, there was no difference in men's and women's success rates, but when they assessed the primary scientist on the application, men fared much better than women.

In hospital settings, studies have shown that women are less likely to have their pain taken seriously, and are often given less pain relief compared with men.

The lack of interest in our very different bodies means that we're being overlooked in all fields, not just the menopause.

CHAPTER TWO

The Knowledge:
A Road Map of Menopause

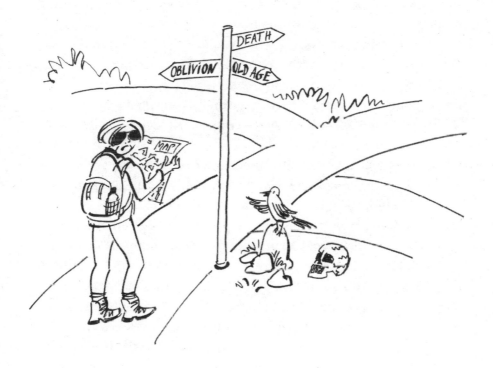

'So, how do we find out what to do about it?
There is currently no clear path to illumination.'

The starting post: the science

What is the menopause? Well, for all the secrecy and overtones of doom, it's a pretty straightforward concept, and directly connected to its younger sister, puberty. First the hormones go up, and then, decades later, they go down again.

'The most eggs you have is when you are a five-month-old foetus. Female babies are born with around two million eggs in their ovaries, and we only (only!) have four to five hundred periods in our lifetime, one a month for around forty years,' explains our menopause expert, Dr Tonye Wokoma, consultant in community gynaecology, sexual and reproductive health, in Hull.

'These die off at a rate of ten thousand or so a month pre-puberty and then a thousand or so afterwards. At puberty, the pituitary gland in the brain releases follicle-stimulating hormone (FSH). This messages the ovaries and tells them to start ripening an egg within a follicle, which produces oestrogen to prepare the womb lining,' says Tonye.

'Next, luteinising hormone (LH) from the pituitary gland informs the ovaries it's time to release the egg into the fallopian tubes. The empty follicle becomes what's called the corpus luteum, which produces oestrogen and progesterone.' As we all know, the egg/hormone business is cyclical, occurring around every twenty-eight to thirty-five days.

'The ovaries make three hormones: oestrogen, progesterone and testosterone. There are oestrogen receptors around our body, from our reproductive systems, to our hearts, bones, skin and brain. Progesterone maintains the lining of the womb and testosterone is vital for the growth, maintenance and repair of the reproductive tissues as well as libido, mood, bones and strength. Should the egg not be fertilized, the womb lining is shed, and you have a period.'

> The moment itself, going 'through' the menopause – how can you possibly know that it's the last time an egg will plop into the fallopian tube? – will probably go unnoticed and unmarked. It's all about the years before and after.

Puberty still has its mysteries, but it's far more heavily investigated than menopause. It is also a celebrated rite of passage, mostly famed for the moodiness, spots, parent loathing and door slamming that all kicks off when the sex hormones get the business of fertility underway. Behaviourally, I'd say that it puts menopausal women in the clear, or maybe we've just learned better restraint by mid-life!

Menopause isn't a nice and tidy stopping of the menstrual cycle. 'When you get towards the age of menopause, your eggs are starting to run out, so it's not as easy for the ovaries to produce one every month,' explains Tonye. 'The body becomes more resistant to FSH, so this goes up to try and get the ovaries to work. If you're not taking hormones, in the form of the pill, for example, cycles can become shorter and periods closer together or more irregular. The other hormones begin to fluctuate, and that's when women start to experience symptoms.' The perimenopause is, she says with restraint, a bit chaotic.

Surprisingly, during these years, oestrogen may rise, or spike, by as much as thirty per cent,[1] before it finally plummets.

'Gradually the ovaries stop producing these three hormones in sufficient quantities and go to sleep,' continues Tonye. 'Periods become further spaced and finally stop. Twelve months after your last period, you are said to have gone through the menopause.'

The unmarked path of perimenopause

The puzzling thing about menopause of course is that it's not a direct diagnosis, but a retrospective one. The moment itself, going 'through' the menopause – how can you possibly know that it's the last time an egg will plop into the fallopian tube? – will probably go unnoticed and unmarked. It's all about the years before and after.

It's said that more than eighty per cent of women will have some symptoms before and after the menopausal moment. They may start a few months or years before and last an average of four years after the menopause, but they might be as long as ten years before and twelve years or more after your last period, which adds up to a good quarter of our expected lifespan.[2] Incidentally, the oldest recorded menopause was said to have occurred at the age of 104, which seems both unlikely and a particularly low blow.[3]

The accepted wisdom is that the perimenopause starts in your mid-forties. But the perimenopause is the stealth pilot of the process. Most of us are unaware that the effects of see-sawing hormones may have quietly begun in our early forties or even late thirties.[4] The perimenopause is only now being recognized as a significant marker on our biological journey.

Menopause before the age of forty is called premature menopause or Premature Ovarian Insufficiency (POI). It affects one in every hundred women under the age of forty. Between forty and forty-five, it's called early menopause and will affect five per cent of women. The final curtain for menstruation occurs on average at the age of fifty-one. I was bang on fifty-one, like a school swot.

So, from women in their early forties, who have no idea that burgeoning anxiety may be down to fluctuating oestrogen levels, to women in their mid-sixties being told they *have* to come off HRT, we're not being properly informed.

Initially, as in my case, changes may well be vague, and get gradually worse over time. It can be near impossible to know whether you are perimenopausal, grumpy, ill, overworked, in a bad relationship or stressed and – knowing modern women – with a permanent and overriding sense of guilt that it's entirely, if inexplicably, your fault. That's why ignorance becomes our enemy. Without being aware of what we might be looking for, it can take quite some time to recognize what's actually taking place.

Psychologist and menopause specialist Dr Meg Arroll tells me that women generally access healthcare only when functioning decreases. 'That's the point at which you can't achieve all your activities in daily life. You are overwhelmed. That's why we need public health consolidation. Women wait a long time for help, but once they have a diagnosis and the right treatment, they realize that they've had a few years of feeling lost, and that it didn't have to be that way.'

This is little comfort when you're on your knees with exhaustion and finally make a GP appointment! And, perhaps even more aggravatingly, the moment you near fifty, every emotion you display is likely to be dismissed as being caused by the menopause rather than perfectly justified dismay, displeasure, anger or frustration.

Incidentally, a friend's more enlightened children, having heard us chatting about this book, *are* asking her, repeatedly, whether it 'might be the menopause' if she so much as snaps at them, or forgets where she has put her car keys. 'They are, on the whole, absolutely right,' she says. 'The problem is that I don't want to give them the impression that I am in any way governed by my hormones.'

The mystery of menopause

The menopause is genuinely one of the world's greatest mysteries. Humans are one of only two mammalian species who go through the menopause, the others being various types of whale: orcas, belugas, narwhal and short-finned pilot whales – names which are otherwise helpful only if you take part in very demanding pub quizzes.[5]

The journalist Christa d'Souza also mentions a menopause-enduring aphid in her personal account of menopause, *The Hot Topic*. I have mixed feelings about comparing my biology to that of an insect, though six limbs and the ability to fly would be super useful. As my co-author Alice and I were leaving no stone unturned, we did check this with Professor Simon Leather at the Department of Crop and Environment Science, Harper Adams University, and he says that, while there are a number of aphid species that have a post-reproductive life for which there are a couple of theories, 'I wouldn't actually call it menopause.'[6]

There are all sorts of theories as to the point of an exemption from pregnancy in the second half of our lives. Much of the animal kingdom is destined to procreate from puberty almost to the grave, so we are pretty unusual in our extended post-fertility phase, where we have time to focus on pursuits not determined by our gender. In a still-unexplained diversion from our chimpanzee ancestors, and along with those previously acknowledged whale communities, we are still fit and well enough to live a full life for decades after our last period. Why should that be?

The least inspiring theory is that, historically, once we were unable to have babies, we would probably die anyway. As our baby-making potential came to an end, so did we, assuming we hadn't already expired from blood loss or infection during childbirth itself. But many historians remind us that maximum human lifespan hasn't changed a great deal since classical times; the oft quoted 'three score years and ten' is actually from the Bible. It's just that fewer of us used to achieve that age.[7]

> I have mixed feelings about comparing my biology to that of an insect, though six limbs and the ability to fly would be super useful.

From 1500 to 1800, early church records in the UK suggest that as many as thirty per cent of children died before their fifteenth birthday,[8] and more than a third of women are said to have died during their child-bearing years in medieval times.[9] You needed to survive being born and then avoid smallpox, diphtheria, tuberculosis and whatever other ghastly illnesses took us down before vaccines were invented. If female, you then also needed to pull through the horrors of antibiotic- and anaesthetic-free childbirth on an extremely regular (unplanned) basis, after which point you were reasonably likely to get to old age.

So there will have been plenty of women surviving multiple births and reaching their menopausal years, only to find themselves ridiculed in historical accounts as repulsive, or, in extreme cases, being dunked in a pond or burned at the stake for perceived crimes against the patriarchy.

Grandmother Hypothesis

My favourite explanation of the menopause is also the most likely. What's known as the Grandmother Hypothesis was first put forward in the 1950s. This theory suggests that women have the menopause *because* we are so useful to society in later life.

The pioneering historian, Susan Mattern, argues this very convincingly in her 2019 book, *The Slow Moon Climbs: The Science, History, and Meaning of Menopause.*[10] She points out that, for most mammals, survival of the species depends on generating as many heirs as possible before you die, and the female fertility cycle in those animals has developed to achieve that necessity. But we are different.

She offers some tantalizing clues as to why, contravening the logic of Darwin's natural selection theory, we live way past what's been presumed to be our sex's sole purpose on this earth: that of bearing children. Mattern says that the evidence suggests that we diverged from our closest relatives, the chimpanzees, around six to ten million years ago, and the menopausal phenomenon/our long post-reproductive lifespan presumably occurred more than 130,000 years ago, before we split off from each other to wander the world. 'Menopause occurs in all known human populations'. With today's extended lifespans, many women will have as many years post-fertility as we will have with baby-making potential.

But let's return to our whales, who are a fine example of the Grandmother Hypothesis. Those species who experience a long post-fertility lifespan exist in what are known as matrilineal societies, which means those based on the female rather than the male line. They are made up of small communities headed by a 'grandmother'. This matriarch offers evidence that the foraging, experience and hands-on help with calf-rearing supplied by mature females make their post-reproductive skills of equal value to their procreative.

Although we had dismissed menopause in aphids (see page 30), Professor Leather pointed us in the direction of a study which speculates on their post-reproductive lives. 'A non-reproducing individual could therefore benefit the population by retaining its food-improving ability even when its reproductive function had ceased'.[11] Sounds like the Grandmother Hypothesis again.

In a nutshell, this is what sets us apart from the apes, dogs and cats. Post-menopausal women aren't going to take up time and resources having babies, so they can forage, farm, help raise families or – these days – run global corporations.

Of course, women have always had extensive skills, which have been largely dismissed. The nine-thousand-year-old skeleton of a huntress was discovered during a 2020 archaeological dig in Peru.[12] This hugely challenged the previously held theory that men were the hunters and women the gatherers. Women have of course been hampered to some degree by the fact that men can't have babies. Happily, these days we have nurseries, schools and options for childcare that include fathers, so menopausal women are more likely to be expending their usefulness at work and in wider society, rather than tending to families.

Those of us who are indebted to our mothers, mothers-in-law or an older relative for helping out with childcare, as I am, will particularly relate to the Grandmother Hypothesis. Those of you who *are* grandmothers, and now realize that you are vital to the survival of the human race, may be rethinking your free babysitting policy and considering some sort of minibreak.

The Grandmother Hypothesis, argues Matten, is one of the key reasons humans were able to evolve successfully. Imagine this! Old women are useful! Hold the front page . . . though, not likely. I'm sure there are those who will cry, 'Fie to such a feminine conspiracy theory!' But this is no speculative stab at a thesis, it's an anthropological conclusion based on compelling scientific evidence. Women are as valuable post-menopause as we were before. We know it. Now we just need society to catch up with the idea.

Evolution is all about survival, and that's why menopause might be doing us and future generations a favour healthwise. Susan Bewley, Emeritus Professor (Honorary) of Obstetrics and Women's Health at King's College London, points out that later-life pregnancy is dangerous to women because of our natural ageing process.[13] By preventing us from getting pregnant and dying in childbirth at an advanced age, menopause is a genius result.

She references the Grandmother Hypothesis. 'Live mothers are needed to get their offspring to survive into adulthood. They can also help care for the grandchildren. So, although it seems a bit para-doxical, a shorter reproductive lifespan thanks to the menopause may have given us reproductive advantage,' she says. 'As a species, we have to put so much work into postnatal childcare (given the long years of dependence – unlike other animals) because of our post-birth brain development.'

> The Grandmother Hypothesis, argues Matten, is one of the key reasons humans were able to evolve successfully. Imagine this! Old women are useful! Hold the front page . . .

Either way, nature most definitely wants to keep us alive, even if society considers us redundant. It's a conundrum. The fact that our fertility does decline as we age is frequently argued as being a sexist point, and that women should be allowed to have babies at any time of life. But maybe we should start seeing our infertile later years less as a punishment and more as a gift? Clearly, having choice is important, but we can't deny our biology.

The information maze

We know what the menopause is, and why it may occur. So, how do we find out what to do about it? There is currently no clear path to illumination. My contemporaries may remember the slender books about sex and pregnancy handed to us by our mums in our early teens, probably rather furtively, back in the Seventies and Eighties, less so – I gather – in these more enlightened times.

I certainly wasn't aware of a step-by-step introduction to the menopause, with easy-to-follow diagrams, but I'd be hugely grateful if my daughter was given one. For women now approaching or in the throes of menopause, knowledge is essential. Equally, for young girls, preparation for what's to come counts as an essential part of the toolkit for life.

Until recently, there's been no sense that women need any sort of literature or chat about the end of our fertility, even though it's just as significant a process as the beginning. How has this happened, and especially in a world where we now talk openly about breast cancer, periods and our sex lives (to a greater or lesser degree)? You'd think that an automatic perimenopause GP meeting in your mid-thirties or early forties would be an obvious and positive step. It's certainly part of what we should be asking for, in terms of a new, enlightened approach to women's health, not just in regard to fertility, but all the decades beyond.

There's a strong genetic component; you are very likely to follow your mother in terms of both timing and severity of symptoms.[14] But this information may be extremely hard to extract. We polled a number of friends in their forties and fifties whose mothers – untruthfully, in most cases, we suspect – claim to have no memory of the menopause at all, or point out that in 'their day' you just got on with it and 'there wasn't all this fuss'.

In order to self-diagnose, you first of all need to have somehow absorbed the information that your anxiety, sleepless nights, forgetfulness and irritability, hot flushes and aching joints might be signs of the menopause and not be down to stress, depression, terminal illness or incipient madness.

Next, you will probably go on Dr Google (and discover you have symptoms synonymous with incurable cancer or a rare tropical disease), then phone a friend, or make a doctor's appointment, and at that point you enter the health lottery as to whether you get clear medical advice, a prescription for antidepressants, or an opinion about HRT based entirely on the GP's opinion rather than medical science.

In a 2020 survey of more than one and a half thousand women by Mumsnet and Gransnet, thirty-six per cent of those who sought help from their GP for perimenopause symptoms, and twenty-six per cent of those who sought help for menopause symptoms, say they visited their GP three times or more before being prescribed appropriate medication or help.[15]

'I don't rate HRT' is a doctor's response that I've heard from so many women now that I can't dismiss it as being anything but commonplace. Am I alone in not caring whether they rate it or not, so long as my basic right to have it prescribed is fulfilled?

The muddle of medical training

I had no idea that end-of-menses education wasn't a key part of clinical training for our medics, until it became relevant to me. I get the impression that, for the most part, it's not so much ignored as just mentioned too briefly.

Fortunately, there are such groups as the British Menopause Society (BMS), who are doing a sterling job producing information for clinicians and patients, as well as running menopause courses, with around one and a half thousand people attending every year.

'The British Menopause Society continues to address the issues facing menopause service delivery by actively encouraging, promoting and providing education to GPs as well as clinicians in secondary care,' says the chairman, consultant gynaecologist Haitham Hamoda.

'In contrast to other European countries, where regular health checks may take place in the absence of a particular clinical problem, the UK does not operate the same preventative structure. This applies to most clinical areas, not just the menopause. There are limitations on the current provision of menopause care as a result of the latter, but the British Menopause Society has never accepted the status quo as being how menopause care should be delivered.'

I asked menopause counsellor Diane Danzebrink,[16] creator of the national #MakeMenopauseMatter campaign and the not-for-profit organization Menopause Support, whether training was really as arbitrary as it seemed. Diane has been fighting the lack of standard menopause education across the medical profession since 2015.

When I was asked to go into the local medical school to teach a revision session to second-year medical students, I assumed that they would have a good basic level of knowledge, but I was shocked when it quickly became clear, as we talked, that they knew very little. When I asked how much menopause education they have received, I was told they had flicked through a few slides.

What many recently trained GPs tell you is that they learned almost nothing about menopause during their training. Historically, society and medicine have been male dominated. That has resulted in gender bias which affects many aspects of women's health. It is worth remembering that not even all gynaecologists have good menopause knowledge, and in its ninety-year history there have only ever been two female presidents of the Royal College of Obstetricians and Gynaecologists, so it's really no surprise that menopause has been overlooked and poorly served.

In May, 2021, Menopause Support asked medical schools about their menopause provision. 41 percent of the 32 (out of 33) schools who responded didn't have a mandatory education programme for their students. Many universities said that they expected students to gain menopause education whilst on GP training placements. As Diane says, 'It is both tragic and disgraceful that women are still frequently failed, when they are dismissed, offered antidepressants or sent off on a round of referrals to rheumatology, cardiology and sometimes psychiatry, costing the NHS valuable time and money and causing needless distress to women. Better menopause education is clearly a win/win situation, but we need action, not words, from those in positions to effect long overdue change.'

Many GPs feel equally strongly about the subject. Dr May Jay is an NHS GP working in the West Midlands, and is very direct about it. 'I had no adequate training in menopause at all when I was studying medicine in the early 2000s. In our gynaecology rotation, we learned about the hormonal cycle in women and attended one menopause clinic. That was it. We were given little specialist booklets for each rotation. The GP one had five pages about the menopause and that was our only point of reference.' She says that she feels she knew very little until she needed to prescribe HRT for the first time. 'In addition, over the last decade, I've learned that the spectrum of "normal" is very broad when it comes to menopause. I feel strongly that we need to give women credit; explain treatment options and allow them to weigh up the pros and cons and make their own decisions as to what they'd like to do. Personally, I very much recommend HRT, but because of the perceived risk, some doctors are reluctant.' (See Chapter Four for more on HRT.)

I need to point out, by the way, that I am in no way denigrating the medical profession. They have plenty to deal with in an underfunded and overstretched NHS, and they're doing a brilliant job in countless ways. Many GPs and practice nurses are, without question, beacons of information and excellence when it comes to menopause. But not all. A rethink in training on this period of women's lives, and one which is costing the NHS a fortune because of misdiagnosis, not to mention the cost to women's long-term health and mental well-being, would seem imperative in the twenty-first century.

Then there are such pioneers as Dr Louise Newson; mentioned as a matter of course in almost every menopause article written, a bit like Colin Firth as Mr Darcy in any Top Ten Iconic Movie Moments. 'Traditionally, menopause education for women has been done by gynaecologists, which in my mind is wrong,' she says. 'Education should come from GPs and nurses who understand that the menopause is a long-term hormone deficiency with health risks rather than just something causing a few hot flushes!'

Dr Newson has created an evidence-based menopause programme for GPs which allows doctors to achieve appraisals remotely via UK company Fourteen Fish.[17] 'We can access thousands of doctors very quickly. Women are more empowered about the menopause, but doctors are less so, and this needs to change.' Her website, menopausedoctor.co.uk, has been adopted by the Royal College of GPs (RCGP), whose official educational library is aimed at patients and healthcare professionals wishing to learn more about the menopause.

A motorway of misinformation

Going to the GP with feelings of anxiety might be construed as many things. Which is, I'd argue, why it's necessary that all women need to know such feelings may well be indicative of falling oestrogen and not mental illness.

This brings me to another gaping hole in the currently available information. One of the biggest medical scandals in history occurred in 2002, when a study was halted on the basis that HRT significantly increased the risk of breast cancer (I'm paraphrasing here, as we delve into it in depth in later chapters; see page 83).[18] This led to Hormone Replacement Therapy (HRT), the greatest and most effective tool we have in managing the majority of menopausal symptoms, being branded as dangerous for well over a decade. Over half the women taking it stopped, and it's only now being correctly credited and used for rebalancing plummeting hormones.

Following that study (and various others around the time), debate raged over whether or not you were taking your life in your hands by succumbing to HRT. The NICE guidance – which is to say, the official guidelines – was reconsidered and rewritten in 2015 to include HRT,[19] but the damage had been done. From 2002 onwards, if you took HRT and then developed breast cancer, you might suffer the added burden of wondering whether it was your fault.

The rocky road of injustice

Quality of treatment for the menopause depends to some extent on where you live and your cultural background. I knew that menopause had an image problem, but it's far worse than I thought. Here, any sense of fairness grinds to an abrupt halt.

Buckinghamshire-based family GP, Dr Nighat Arif, specializes in women's health and is a passionate menopause campaigner. She says that menopause globally is perceived as a white, affluent, middle-class condition. 'Look at the literature in the UK. Do you ever see a Black or Indian woman in the pictures? I told my mother that she was probably going through the menopause when she was fifty-six, and she dismissed me: "It's a white woman's disease".'

This means that ethnic minorities – Asian, Black, Chinese and Arab women – aren't given enough consideration, and research and funding into their needs and experiences is appallingly low. 'If you don't look at posters or pamphlets and see yourself, how can you relate? That, in turn, means women are missing out on seeking treatment and therefore receiving potentially life-saving medication,' says Nighat.

'I am currently treating the Afro-Caribbean and Pakistani women who came off HRT during the 2002 scandal, and are now suffering from osteoporosis and cardiovascular problems,' she says. 'It was entirely preventable in these high-risk groups, and it breaks my heart.'

Different cultures experience or describe different symptoms. For White women, the classic sign of menopause is the hot flush, but if you are Pakistani, it is more likely to be described as sleeplessness

– which can be affiliated to night sweats, but isn't interpreted as such – palpitations and head-to-toe pain. Nighat does a lot of documenting: 'In our language – Urdu – palpitations translates as "my heart is beating fast". Many women describe they feel a "heart sinking", but when I say "depression", they disagree. I've concluded that it's anxiety and depression combined.'

In global studies, it has been noted that Japanese women tend to complain more of shoulder stiffness and general fatigue,[20] and Nighat has seen Turkish women mentioning eye problems rather than hot flushes. 'I ask Arab women how bad their hot flushes are, and they say, "Imagine standing in the Dubai desert." As ever, there is no one size fits all!'

Although the standard age is given as fifty-one, a 2011 study reminded that Black and Latina women are more likely to reach menopause at forty-nine, and a 2015 study revealed that African-American women suffered from hot flushes for an average of 10.1 years and Chinese women for 5.4 years. It has been repeatedly pointed out that there is both racial bias in discussing menopause, and far less research into the Black experience.[21]

There is also a reluctance to speak about it in some communities. 'I hear some women saying that they feel ashamed, concerned that they are infertile and worried that their husband might be looking for a second marriage – this is particularly the case in early menopause.'

And finally, there are linguistic barriers. 'There is no word for menopause in Urdu, where women tend to say *banchie* – or barren. Vulva does not exist as a word either, so these terms are entering Urdu.'

Dr May Jay agrees: 'When I was growing up, we simply didn't speak about such things, and although Urdu is my mother tongue, I don't know the words for sex or periods. Although things are more open now, those words haven't developed. I recently had to tell a woman she wasn't ovulating, but in Urdu. She looked utterly shocked, which I assumed was down to the revelation, but when I asked my mother whether I'd explained correctly, she collapsed in laughter. I'd told this poor patient that she wasn't laying eggs.'

Dr Tonye Wokoma points out that some cultures may dismiss the need for medication to treat menopause symptoms. 'This is reflected in their menopause health-seeking behaviours, and they will not access care. There are a lot of myths and misconceptions that surround treatment which frighten women away from seeking help.'

Nighat makes TikTok videos (short films available online) and recorded a podcast in a mixture of Punjabi and Urdu to help Indian and Pakistani women understand the nature of the menopause, and has translated pamphlets about vaginal dryness. The responses she is getting prove the need for information beyond all doubt. Her first TikTok got twenty-six thousand views in a week. 'Millennials are desperate to arm themselves with all the facts, and they're the ones engaging. They can't get the information from their mothers and there's little acknowledgement elsewhere.'

Money paves the way

There's also – as ever – an affluence bias. The poorer the area in which you live, the less likely you are to be offered the medications which could make a difference. A *British Journal of General Practice* paper, using 2018 data, pointed out that in areas of deprivation you were twenty-nine per cent less likely to be prescribed HRT.[22]

'I work in a very deprived area,' says Dr May Jay. 'When I became a GP, I realized that funding isn't fairly allocated. We have the largest area of deprivation in our Clinical Commissioning Group, which decides where funds go, but historically we were paid far less per patient head. By the time people round here access healthcare, they are often very sick. There's fear about taking time off work and about being lectured, as well as there not being the level of education about the importance of seeking help early.'

'I don't think that menopause as a whole, for all women, from all backgrounds, is being dealt with well on the NHS,' says Nighat. 'The wait to see a menopause specialist is extensive and menopause training is not mandatory for all healthcare professionals. So, at the moment, I see little evidence that race, class, culture or concern is addressed.' All the more reason for a professional menopause code of practice when it comes to this unavoidable mid-life experience for all women, no matter their race, colour, financial or cultural position.

The rainbow route

Should you be anything other than a heterosexual, cisgendered (meaning your gender identity matches your sex at birth) woman, there is likely to be an added layer of obtuseness about the menopause.

'Nobody should make assumptions about sexual orientation,' says Annie Cunningham at LGBT Foundation. 'When we are experiencing menopause, in its varying stages, it's a time of vulnerability and confusion for a lot of us, and an underestimated barrier for many is the assumption made by medical professionals about the gender of our partners. Very often there is the assumption that you are heterosexual, have a husband etc. and so the dialogue that you hope to be having is founded on an inaccuracy that can be difficult to deal with.'

For trans men and non-binary people who have a uterus, the menopause experience can be complex, she says. Should a trans man or non-binary person be taking testosterone, they will probably go through menopause with reduced or no symptoms. Should a trans man stop taking testosterone, then he will expect to experience menopause, and finding inclusive medical practices can be a challenge during a potentially traumatic time.

Disability

'Another group of women who are overlooked are women with learning disabilities,' says Dr Tonye Wokoma. 'For example, women with Down's syndrome go through the menopause earlier than the average age, with attendant adverse consequences, but this is often not addressed and the right treatment isn't initiated.'

'There's not enough awareness, education or research into this area,' agrees Dr Laura Nicholson, consultant in learning disability psychiatry for NHS Greater Glasgow and Clyde. 'Most women with learning disabilities will have to deal with menopause, and it can be distressing and stressful for them and carers.'

Light at the end of the tunnel?

It's not all doom and gloom. The #MakeMenopauseMatter campaign goal – for menopause to be taught in secondary education – had already received many thousands of signatures when, in 2019, the then Education Secretary, Damian Hinds, announced that menopause would become part of pupils' sex education in England from September 2020.[23] There are specialist NHS menopause clinics, but these are few and far between.[24] In May 2021, there were 101 British Menopause Society recognized NHS menopause clinics on their register (and 133 private), and that's to treat an estimated thirteen million hot, insomniac, anxious, suffering women. The British Menopause Society has just launched a new menopause programme and is increasing its courses, and, in May 2021, The Menopause Charity – of which I am an official supporter – launched. Founded by Dr Louise Newson, they offered free access for one health professional per GP practice to a Confidence in Menopause course. Within two days, over half of the NHS practices in the UK had signed up. At last, progress.[25]

Ever since the Garden of Eden and its spare-rib fantasy, society has been in denial of the fact that women are not physically lesser beings than men, nor are they made from men's bit parts.

Ever since the Garden of Eden and its spare-rib fantasy, society has been in denial of the fact that women are not physically lesser beings than men, nor are they made from men's bit parts. Women are unique, in our biology and in our symptoms. For way too long we've been regarded as secondary components of human (men's) health, so female-specific conditions, aside from childbirth, in which the whole world has an interest, have been left relatively unexplored. There clearly needs to be more focus, training and a roll-out best-practice policy for this issue, which has the potential to negatively impact the present and future health of all women in mid-life.

Every GP surgery in the land needs at least one Dr Menopause. We are fortunate enough to have all manner of automatic health checks and screenings: cervical smears, bowel and breast cancer checks and the over-forties health checks. But why is menopause not on that latter agenda? Surely it should come with a mandatory menopause update so that we know to recognize symptoms such as sleepless nights or aching joints as a possible first sign of diminishing hormones?

What we do have springing up all over the place is a change in attitude. In the last few years, menopause has landed firmly on the agenda for discussion. And we also have all the brilliant people campaigning for better awareness: Dr Louise Newson, Meg Mathews, Liz Earle, Diane Danzebrink, Dr Nighat Arif, Kate Muir and groups such as The Menopause Charity, MPowered Women, Pausitivity, Henpicked, the politicians taking up the cause and, of course, the British Menopause Society. There are plenty of excellent free sources of information all around, if you only seek them out. There is campaigning for education, laws, workplace acknowledgement and more GP training. There is – in a nutshell – hope.

Dorothy Koomson

BESTSELLING AUTHOR DOROTHY KOOMSON, FORTY-NINE

I know that some women think of the menopause as being
the worst thing in the world and dread it, but I've never had
a perception of this time as being either good or bad. It's
just a stage of life. If you've been taking in the message that
you're no longer young and relevant, then that must be
difficult.

Menopausal women are seen as a bit unstable and mad,
but that's the perception, not the reality. The problem is that
we're still scared to talk about it and admit that we might be
going through it. I've not had expectations, which I think
makes it easier.

My hormones have never been straightforward: from a
very young age I had painful and heavy periods, with tender
breasts, back pain and constipation. About four years ago I
had bleeding in between periods and it was discovered that
this was probably due to a combination of polyps, fibroids,
endometriosis and polycystic ovaries. I ended up having an
ablation – removal of my womb lining, and this hugely
lessened the symptoms for a couple of years.

In 2011, I had some hot flushes, and thought it was the
beginning of the menopause. Other symptoms included
being tired and gaining weight in spite of not eating much,
as well as being cold all the time and dry hair. I went to the
doctor and, after a blood test, it was discovered that I had a
thyroid condition called Hashimoto, an autoimmune disease
causing an underactive thyroid. The doctor told me there
was nothing they could do and, because my thyroid was
working in bursts, I had to wait for it to stop working
completely before they would do anything. I changed my
diet and went gluten free which helped enormously, but after
four years of battling to be taken seriously, I paid to see a
consultant endocrinologist who told me that I should have

been given medication a long time ago. Taking medication made a huge difference, and as there are links between menopausal symptoms and thyroid problems, those symptoms eased as well.

To my surprise, when I started to use an online period tracker a year ago, I realized that my periods are pretty regular. A week before my period I will have the same symptoms: painful breasts, feeling cross, feeling exhausted and lower back pain. The hot flushes still come and go, and the big problem is night sweats – I have them for about a week to ten days before my period and I'll wake up in the morning with my clothes and my bed soaked through. Sometimes I have to get up and get changed in the middle of the night.

I do feel that being somebody who is curious and constantly does research helps when it comes to dealing with such things. It means that I'm not constantly going to my GP, having learned through my Hashimoto experience that you aren't necessarily going to get solutions.

With any research I do, I focus on proper doctors and looking at as many sources as I can, especially when it comes to diet, supplements and lifestyle changes. There are so many people out there who are pushing snake oil – lots of expensive gadgets and concoctions – at women who are arguably in a vulnerable frame of mind, and desperate to hear that one simple thing will change how they feel. I'm always aware of this when I read about anything online – I might just be falling for something because it promises to make everything better in one fell swoop. It's rarely that simple.

In 2020, during the first lockdown, I took up Zoom exercise with a group of friends. Every morning we would do a YouTube class together and I was very disappointed to find that it made me feel so much better! That means I have to keep at it. I also take a range of supplements that concentrate on balancing my gamma-linolenic acid (GLA), vitamin D, iron and magnesium levels, as well as supplements that will balance the levels of 'good' and 'bad' oestrogen in my body. I've found a couple of experts online who give some really good advice because they are advising on my thyroid condition as well as my reproductive health.

I have no plans to try HRT. With all the conditions I have that are usually the result of excess hormones, I don't think adding more will help. Obviously, if there's no other option, then I will look at it again.

I try not to worry about getting older when it comes to my career or lifestyle. I'm very fortunate in that I work mainly for myself and I strive to make each book better. Work-wise, I suppose that my only worry would be that my joints might seize up. But ageing is very much a part of life and I accept it as such. I'm here and can enjoy life in a relatively healthy state of mind and body, so there is no mourning lost fertility for me. The moment it's gone, it's gone, and like every birthday you reach, it's just another part of your life to be moved onto.

Susannah Constantine

WRITER AND BROADCASTER SUSANNAH CONSTANTINE,
FIFTIES

When I was first asked to comment about the menopause, my initial reaction was that there's too much fucking talk about the subject. It's become a bandwagon for some to jump upon or a badge of honour that others want a pat on the back for having survived. It's part of being a woman. It's a life stage. I don't *want* to know about it, and it's not an issue for my daughters. My children (two of whom are daughters) have never thrown a menopausal insult if I've been a bad tempered, erratic old bat. They've never asked me if I'm going through it, and I've been lucky, with no physical symptoms. Why do women want to define themselves by it? It's frankly baffling.

And then I thought about it, and remembered that, from the age of fifty or fifty-one, my chronic anxiety intensified and I didn't even consider it might be the menopause. But it was, because I know that happened between fifty-one and fifty-four.

Then I remembered my friends who have gone through the mill of menopause and had a terrible time. They really suffered. Because my experience – and in retrospect, I'd have loved some HRT – was smooth, I'm not really aware of how bad it can be, or sympathetic.

Finally, I thought about my mother, who had a really awful menopause, and her manic depression and bipolar disorder went into major decline after this period. Perhaps my denial of the subject is a form of self-protection.

We can learn from everyone. I've revised my initial opinion and feel a bit guilty now. We need to learn from and support each other. Nobody ought to feel isolated or alone. It should be a time when we are revered for our wisdom and life experience.

Nobody believed it might be menopause

PROOFREADER CLAIRE ANNALS, FORTY-SIX

I'd been suffering mood swings for three years, since the age of forty, and my periods had become so heavy that for a day a month I was completely unable to leave the house. My GP told me that I was too young to be experiencing the symptoms I described, but there were times when I felt completely out of control, and would be shouting at myself (in my head!) to calm down, because I got into a panic over the tiniest of things. The bleeding continued for two years, during which time I was passing clots the size of fists.

In addition to numerous investigations, I was given painkillers, tranexamic acid (used to clot blood), progesterone tablets and injections called Zoladex, which is also used to treat prostate cancer and helps in the treatment of some breast cancers and endometriosis. Some of the side effects are – ironically – menopausal symptoms. I suffered hot flushes, night sweats, mood swings and unpredictable behaviour, itchy skin and 'furry' tongue with a metallic taste.

Finally, in May 2019, I was given HRT. It was as though a switch had been flicked and I was 'me' again for the first time since I was forty! The bleeding began to lessen and I haven't bled since November 2019. I don't know whether the HRT stopped the bleeding, but it did give me back my happiness.

All along, I have been told that I was too young to be experiencing the menopause, but looking back, my mother was around the same age as me when she started to have symptoms.

I'm repeatedly offered antidepressants

WRITER SARAH HASELWOOD, FORTIES

Around the age of forty-one, I stopped sleeping and developed terrible and crushing anxiety around the time of my periods. I went to see my GP, who suggested antidepressants. I also put on weight around my middle, in spite of exercising a lot and not eating any more than usual. I'd taken antidepressants before, when I suffered a bereavement, and knew that this feeling was very different. I'm now forty-four, and have been to see different GPs three times. They've done investigations, and there's nothing wrong with me, except these symptoms. I asked whether it might be menopause-related and they said no and kept on offering the antidepressants. Eventually, I signed up to a health programme, cut out sugar, increased my fibre intake, did more weight-bearing exercise and Pilates. I feel a little better, but don't feel I've been offered any sort of solution.

Menopause made my taste buds change

BUSINESSWOMAN JANE HALLAM, FIFTY-FOUR

For me, the most bizarre (but by no means the worst) symptom of menopause was my changing taste buds. I had been vegetarian since my twenties, more from taste than principle. Then, aged forty-seven, I went off coffee completely, to the extent that I thought I might be pregnant. Then I started to crave baked salmon, which isn't something I've ever eaten much of. Gradually, my cravings extended to meat: black pudding and mince. Now, five years later, I am a fully fledged carnivore again. I've no idea why it happened, but wonder whether it's something to do with my body needing extra protein.

It's a lot of fuss

AUTHOR LIZ HODGKINSON, SEVENTIES

Brought up as I was on dire tales of women going mad and behaving like crazy old witches after the menopause, I spent my adult life dreading it.

But when it actually happened, it was nothing like that. I had been on the pill for many years and, in my late forties, when it was unlikely I would ever become pregnant again, I stopped taking it and waited for the menopause to happen.

Now, should I take HRT or wait for some symptoms? I decided on the latter and to let nature take its course. As it was, I'm glad I did, as I experienced only one awful event, aged just over fifty. I had just returned from the theatre with my then-partner when I started to bleed heavily, getting through fourteen tampons in about an hour.

My partner called for an ambulance, as I felt I was bleeding to death, and I was admitted to hospital for a D and C, which removes the lining of the womb. The gynaecologist, who looked about twelve, told me it was the start of the menopause and decided against the op, prescribing a couple of doses of progesterone instead. She also prescribed iron tablets, as the flooding had made me anaemic.

I went home the same day, the bleeding dried up and that was it, basically. I had no more symptoms, no hot flushes, no weight gain, and never took HRT or, indeed, any other menopausal remedy. Not a single one of the supposedly awful side effects of the menopause happened to me.

And I have not gone mad, although that may be for other people to judge. One of my friends, also going through the menopause at the same time, reckoned we were talking so much we didn't even notice it.

Now, more than twenty-five years after that single event, I remain perfectly healthy. So am I just lucky, or normal? My view is that the menopause is a natural event, not an illness, and if you can get through it without medical intervention, so much the better, and my guess is that around eighty per cent of women get through it without any major problems at all.

Just knowing what it was helped with symptoms

UPCYCLING/SEWING SOCIAL ENTREPRENEUR
KEMI OLOYEDE, FIFTIES

African women are traditionally superstitious in certain ways. If there are specific health traits or conditions in the family, by saying it and discussing it, it's affirmation and confirmation and also lets it take root. So, for example, menopause wasn't discussed in our house. Culturally, that means that you may not learn about important life events. There's also the fact that my mother's generation simply didn't discuss what were seen as intimate problems so much. But, had I known, I wouldn't have panicked once it did start.

I was told about the birds and bees in the most vague way: if you go near a boy, you get pregnant. But I look back, and there was a period when Mum was lethargic due to the hot flushes. I remember her putting the fan on the whole time.

In my family, we have babies into our fifties, so, even aged fifty, when I was four years into perimenopause, Mum was suggesting that I have another baby. Around the age of forty-six, I started feeling very lethargic and just not present. I also had terrible palpitations. As I was teaching at the time, I thought that it might be work stress. I was sent for an ECG, which was fine, but, while chatting to the nurse and discussing my other symptoms – bad skin, breakouts for the first time in my life, and poor hair condition – she asked about my periods, which were irregular. 'It might be the beginning of the menopause,' she said.

The hot flushes became really intense by the age of fifty. They've gone down tremendously, but there was a time when I had the fan on almost constantly in the evening.

Just the other day, a friend and I were wondering how on earth our mothers knew about this time of our lives but didn't ever discuss it with us! I am going through it now, and I'd like to think that, if I had a daughter, I'd flag it up.

CHAPTER THREE

First Impact

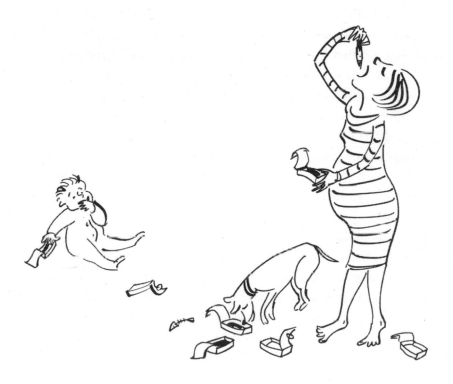

'... three months of oily fish addiction, which on more than one
occasion resulted in my husband returning home to find
his baby girl crawling the floor while her mother sat
with sardine can in hand like a guilty addict ...'

The symptoms

One of the major challenges with menopause, from peri to post, is that nobody can tell you when it starts or stops. Who in their fifties can recall with any accuracy when they last had their period? Most of us won't recognize the historical day until months later. This makes it difficult for anyone wanting to mourn or celebrate the final passing of their periods with any accuracy. Those intent on performing a ritual or holding a festival for stopped periods will probably find it's a date as hard to pin down as an MP elaborating on a personal sex scandal.

Pinpointing when the decline begins is equally difficult, in spite of the fact that the time to address and even treat the symptoms of health-impairing drops in oestrogen levels is likely to be in our mid-forties, or even sooner. The average age of perimenopause is said to be forty-five,[1] but as I've pointed out, many of us may experience symptoms before this moment. Even if you are on red alert, identifying this stage can be hard. A lack of oestrogen affects the entire body and brain, and there are tens of potential symptoms, but they are entirely subjective. No two women will have the same experience, and many of the indicators aren't necessarily associated with menopause, such as thinning hair and dry skin. I now know that there might be at least thirty ways of recognizing your hormonal variations. Many websites cite thirty-four, which is now an oft-quoted number. Others say, rather vaguely, that there are 'more than one hundred'.[2]

Of course there are the hot flushes, those sweaty, fanning-yourself-by-an-open-window menopausal clichés, which are a pretty obvious sign of hormones going off kilter. But the first subtle indications of declining hormones and the crepuscular days of fertility go unrecognized by the majority of us, for whom the aforementioned and ubiquitous hot flush is the only marker given as a reliable warning signal that biological changes are afoot.

But, in addition to the overheating, irregular periods and night sweats, you might – or might not – suffer from joint pain, insomnia, tender breasts, brain fog, irritability, depression, anxiety, dry skin, itchy skin, acne, thinning hair, loss of libido, fatigue, burning mouth, gum problems, weight gain (especially increased fat around your middle), bloating, headaches, vaginal dryness, incontinence, increased body odour, thyroid problems, increased bruising, tinnitus and palpitations. What a hoot, and that list is by no means exhaustive. I have friends who have referenced such random and obscure ailments as swollen eyes, boiling hot feet (but no other body part!), itchy scalps and numbness in their extremities as being linked to their hormones.

There's some comfort afforded by that plentiful list. It makes it less shameful that I entered my own menopausal moment unequipped with any of the knowledge I'm now enthusiastically sharing, and is probably why I've embarked on a 'survivor's guide' with all the evangelical glee of a new convert.

I am well aware that my experiences are only the tip of the menopausal iceberg, or – more aptly – the summit of the simmering volcano that signals that our bodies are rebooting. There are many women out there who won't suffer so much as one hot flush, but who'll experience anxiety or anger, exhaustion, feel horny or lack libido entirely, will endure crippling headaches or weight gain, become dehydrated from head to toe at the same time as they are conversely awash in sweat, lose hair in some places and gain it in less welcome areas. Confused? You definitely will be!

> I am well aware that my experiences are only the tip of the menopausal iceberg, or – more aptly – the summit of the simmering volcano that signals that our bodies are rebooting.

My experience

It's easy for me to sit here typing away today, advising you to keep an eye on your biological clock long before it stops ticking. I have the smug satisfaction of having fumbled my way through the tunnel and emerged, blinking and triumphant on the other side. The good news is, as we wake up to the toxic propaganda around this most natural of processes, it doesn't actually need to be a dark enclosed space at all.

It's likely that having spent my early forties making babies, I missed the worst ailments of the latter part of that decade, when many women's symptoms start to manifest.

Rather, in a positive pile-up of female reproductive activity, I managed to produce two children and traverse through menopause all in the same decade. It's a scenario in which I should imagine increasing numbers of women are finding themselves, as, in the Western world, we frequently embark on motherhood perilously late. While the full stop of fertility remains steadfast at around fifty for most of us, the ability to get pregnant naturally diminishes from our thirties, and especially our mid-thirties. I make no apologies for mentioning this, by the way. It is a biological fact that it's harder to conceive as you get older.[3]

To digress, but hopefully informatively, pregnancy, even in my early forties, which is when I had my two children, was, unlike the next phase in my biological evolution, actually a pleasure. After an emotionally wearing and erotically dwindling twelve-month period trying to conceive, I sailed through the first gestation without incident and gave birth to a healthy little girl called Molly Mae. My son, Dan, born thirteen months later, was a surprise to us all, conceived just five months after his sister was born.

My first child seems to have provided the reproductive stimulation my body needed for round two, and possibly beyond, had I wanted to carry on down that route. My second outing, apart from three months of oily fish addiction, which on more than one occasion resulted in my husband returning home to find his baby girl crawling the floor while her mother sat with sardine can in hand like a guilty addict, was otherwise also relatively uneventful. In fact, using my favourite bible, *What To Expect When You're Expecting*,[4] there were few surprises that weren't detailed in that wonderful week-on-week companion to gestation.

Sadly, such predictability is not characteristic of the menopause trek. Perhaps it's because I had the two experiences of birth and menopause so close together that I am so acutely aware of the yawning chasm that exists between them in terms of knowing what to expect.

Molly was only six years old when I started to experience the first hints of diminishing egg quality, but I had no idea that they were hormone related because I simply didn't have the information. If only the course of a woman's menopause were as predictable as that of carrying a baby – without diminishing the unique experience – and there were such easy-to-read and clearly diagrammed books as those available for pregnancy. I'd love to see 'irritability' or 'low libido' depicted as a medical diagram.

My own initial menopausal symptoms weren't anything I might have been expecting even if I had been better clued up. They became noticeable at the age of forty-nine, and I then went through two years of low-level anxiety and high-level insomnia before I finally had a diagnosis, and then, through HRT, supplements and deep breathing, some respite.

Below are some of the main symptoms. Our menopause specialist Dr Tonye Wokoma gives brief solutions, many of which we investigate in more depth in later chapters.

Periods (of Change)

A good clue as to the state of your hormones is your periods, which are likely to become irregular; initially they may get closer together and then further apart, which is what happened to me. You may start to suffer PMT out of the blue or find existing PMT is worse, and bleeding can be far heavier as the womb lining builds up more between periods, or it may be lighter. Discharge may change in colour and quantity. A 2014 multi-ethnic SWAN study of 1,320 mid-life women (African American, White, Chinese and Japanese) showed that ninety-one per cent recorded between one and three occurrences, in a three-year period, of bleeding that lasted ten or more days, and seventy-eight per cent recorded three or more days of heavy flow.[5]

> ***Tonye says:*** Heavy periods can be treated with a hormone coil, which is a first line NICE[6] treatment, or the contraceptive pill (both combined pill or progestogen-only pill) and non-steroidal anti-inflammatory drugs (NSAIDs) such as ibuprofen. It is important that, if periods are a problem, they are assessed by a GP to exclude something more sinister. Women have often gained weight, and making lifestyle changes such as improving your diet and doing extra exercise may help. Obesity is a known risk factor for many cancers, including endometrial and breast cancer, as well as other health conditions. Endometrial cancer often presents with abnormal or post-menopausal bleeding.

Worrisome Times

Having never suffered from it before, I was completely thrown by my debilitating and irrational anxiety. I had little to be genuinely stressed about, and yet there was no respite, and no filter.

I'd be as agitated about the online groceries as I was about getting home from the USA in time to relieve the babysitter. I just assumed that I needed to cope and get on with it, rather than wondering whether there might be a reason for my generally sensible self to regularly disintegrate into a seething mass of panic over what – rationally – I knew to be very little, in the scheme of things. For someone accustomed to seeing the larger picture, and generally able to rise above ill humour or irritability in order to get things done, this was frustrating and upsetting.

> I'd be as agitated about the online groceries as I was about getting home from the USA in time to relieve the babysitter.

In fact, there was nothing special about my anxiety. It's said that fifty per cent of women may experience mood changes during the menopause, and that's very hard to pin down as a tangible 'symptom', so you are highly unlikely to enjoy the sight of your GP sitting back in her swivel chair and nodding sagely before scribbling a cure-all prescription.[7]

Tonye says: HRT, CBT, mindfulness and meditation may all help, and women should be assessed to see whether antidepressants or anti-anxiety medication might be needed; this may be more likely if you have a past history of depression (including post-natal depression).

Temper Temper

My temperature didn't initially soar. Instead, it was my temper that escalated to the same unbearable heights as my contemporaries' body-heat. My teenage daughter insists that during this period I once threw a book at her! Luckily (if it actually happened) I missed, and, like childbirth, it's a moment I've happily forgotten, although it will doubtless feature, in a couple of decades' time, when she skewers me with her misery memoir of childhood with an agony aunt.

What I do remember is two years of utter confusion and despair, wondering who the harpy in the house was and why it was, if my heart rate was any indication, that even I was scared of her. Horror films about serial killers suffering terrifying divergent personalities (from *Psycho* to *Split*) briefly became an exercise in empathy as I experienced what it feels like when you become a total stranger to yourself. I think all women, however easy their periods have been, can empathize with the sensation of out-of-control hormones. Imagine feeling like you do the day before your period, but most of the time.

I found a study that I thought was highly amusing, suggesting that, for seventy per cent of menopausal women, irritability is the main mood symptom. The researchers were trying to establish what they called a 'new, female-specific irritability rating scale' and what most of us would call 'stating the bleeding obvious'.[8]

> ***Tonye says:*** HRT, CBT, mindfulness and meditation. Proper assessment is needed and a holistic approach should be taken, looking at sleeping, stress, family situation and whether lifestyle changes might help.

Hot or Not

When you have a hot flush (vasomotor symptoms), they're like nothing else. Mostly I was spared. I had the sum total of two, but I'll never forget the speed and strength of the heat that traversed from my feet to my head in a matter of seconds, making me feel like a latter-day Joan of Arc just as her ordeal at the stake began.

The hot flush is of course the classic and clichéd menopause symptom, and the one most likely to get you taken seriously. They are actually to do with the oestrogen/brain connection. The part of the brain that controls temperature is called the hypothalamus. When oestrogen levels go down, this becomes very sensitive to changes in body temperature and tries to cool you down via a hot flush – it's like internal central heating gone wrong. As anyone who has suffered a hot flush knows, this is utterly counterproductive, as you actually become scorchingly hot. As many as eighty per cent of us may get them.

I may only have had two minor (in the scheme of things) hot flushes, hardly enough to recognize as a recurring condition, but they were memorable for giving me the unpleasant sensation that someone had dropped me on a bonfire. The best way of describing a hot flush is like someone has removed the soles of your feet and is shooting boiling hot air up through your body, with what feels like the full power of an erupting volcano. It's quite unbelievable, and the extreme heat hits like a physical force. Of course I suspected that they might be connected to the menopause, but then dismissed the idea because they simply weren't regular enough. And also, I was very busy, and I forgot. To those of you suffering on a daily basis, I think this proves that mine really weren't that bad.[9]

Night sweats are the dark sisters of the hot flush, and they can ruin both sleep and quality of life. They occur for the same reason as hot flushes, but with the added indignity and inconvenience of occurring at night-time.

> ***Tonye says:*** Adopt lifestyle changes such as less coffee, smoking, alcohol and spicy food, which may be triggers. Try practical solutions such as fans in offices and bedrooms and wearing natural fibres at night. CBT can help. HRT is the first-line choice, and then there are antidepressants such as paroxetine, citalopram or fluoxetine, venlafaxine and anticonvulsants such as gabapentin. Or clonidine (a drug used to treat raised blood pressure in the past) is licensed for use with hot flushes, but there can sometimes be side effects such as dry eyes and a dry mouth. The British Menopause Society and other professional bodies state that SSRIs (Selective Serotonin Reuptake Inhibitors) should not be offered for vasomotor symptoms unless HRT cannot be given.

Sleep Free

It's hardly surprising that I was ill tempered, as I was also distraught from lack of sleep. Every night I woke with a start at three a.m. and didn't really sink back into oblivion again. Finding reason was no longer in my skill set; as my stress levels escalated, my nights were elongated by my inability to sleep, and my days disappeared in a haze of exhaustion while I tried to combine work and childcare.

At first I thought my sleeplessness was caused by my inability to deal with the demands of parenting two rapidly growing young children, and working as well.

Women's tendency to blame themselves doesn't help at all when it comes to the often-vague nature of menopausal symptoms. Rather than wondering whether there might be a medical cause for my lack of sleep, I simply resorted to the conclusion that I wasn't coping. And rather than seeking a solution, I just kept on going, partly because that's what we're expected to do by society, and partly because I had no choice.

We cover this in detail in chapter nine, which is devoted to sleep (see page 217), but most women will suffer some degree of sleep disturbance during the menopausal years.

> ***Tonye says:*** Try HRT, meditation, mindfulness and sleep hygiene in the bedroom: it should be cool, dark and with no screens. Melatonin is available on the NHS to the over fifty-fives.

Be Still My Beating Heart

Palpitations may occur when oestrogen drops, and they sometimes happen during a hot flush. Now, I wouldn't say I suffered from them *per se*. But, once awake at night, I frequently found my heart beating like a rat-tatting machine gun. And of course one of the biggest fears at night is that you are going to have a heart attack and die alone.[10]

> ***Tonye says:*** Palpitations often lead to an underlying sense of dread, panic and anxiety. If you have concerns then see your GP, and if you think you are having a heart attack, call an ambulance. Look at coffee and alcohol consumption, don't smoke, and try relaxation techniques such as mindfulness and meditation.

Memory Matters

The inability to remember simple things, like the names of acquaintances, drove me to distraction. The brain fog of menopause is beyond frustrating, as you lose the ability to bring certain words to the forefront of your mind or have a blank space where there ought to be a meeting. But it's often down to simple chemistry. Oestrogen and testosterone are both vital for memory and concentration.

Again – and I have only learned this, and found myself part of a wide, if vague, sorority, in the course of writing this book – it's incredibly common. Some reports suggest that as many as sixty per cent of women experience some form of memory issue around menopause. A 2013 study into the phenomenon, 'Cognition in Perimenopause',[11] showed that women in the first year of postmenopause performed less well in verbal learning, verbal memory and motor function than those in the earlier stages.

I've relied on mental agility more than many, as I work on live radio, and lapsing into blank spaces when I'm counting on recall is terrifying. So too is having to return to the house five times in order to remember everything I need, or popping out to the shops and returning with everything but the item I went there to buy.

My job at Times Radio relies entirely on quick responses, and short-term recall of salient facts. These days, my pre-programme notes are a forest-worth of illegible scribbles, as I jot down every thought, word or phrase I might need to draw on later. We joke about becoming vague in our old age, but in reality nobody finds it remotely funny. For previously swift and reliable recollection to diminish when you reach your mid to late forties can be utterly alarming and discombobulating (I use the word mainly to prove that things do get better and vocabulary doesn't vanish forever!).

> For previously swift and reliable recollection to diminish when you reach your late forties can be utterly alarming and discombobulating (I use the word mainly to prove that things do get better and vocabulary doesn't vanish forever!).

This means that far too many middle-aged women panic that they are showing early signs of dementia or that they're heading for nervous breakdown. I know I worried about both. In fact, we just need to know that brain fog is frustrating but entirely normal, and that we might benefit from a top-up of oestrogen, testosterone, more sleep, less stress or just a simple recognition that our feelings are entirely normal, if unwelcome, to help alleviate the horror of thinking that our marbles are rolling out of the jar.

Tonye says: HRT can help with brain fog. Tiredness also plays a part, and a healthy diet, proper sleep and exercise make a huge difference.

Feeling Down

All feelings of depression around the time of menopause must be taken seriously. I am so grateful that I didn't suffer from this, but many women do.

As I've already mentioned, your GP may – often erroneously – prescribe antidepressants as a first port of call, and I was staggered at the number of women whose doctors refused to even contemplate a hormonal link between low mood and their age.

We know that brain chemistry can affect mood during this period. In 2014, researchers at the Centre for Addiction and Mental Health at Campbell Family Mental Health Research Institute in Toronto, Canada, identified elevated levels of a brain protein linked to depression, called monoamine oxidase A (MAO-A), in perimenopausal women.[12] They suggested that this might help explain rates of first-time depression at this time. MAO-A (anyone else thinking about those Haribo sweets, Maoams?) is the enzyme that breaks down serotonin, norepinephrine and dopamine – the so-called happy chemicals. High levels of MAO-A have previously been linked to depressive disorders such as postnatal depression. In brain scans, this chemical was on average thirty-four per cent higher in perimenopausal women than in younger women, and sixteen per cent higher in perimenopausal women than in those in menopause.

There is also a link between menopause and suicide, which the

New York Post has called the 'life-threatening side-effect of menopause'.[13] Professor Mary Jane Minkin, clinical professor in the Department of Obstetrics, Gynaecology and Reproductive Sciences at the Yale University School of Medicine, says, 'Perimenopause and menopause precipitate depression in many women, particularly in women who have previously suffered from depression, including post-partum depression and premenstrual dysphoric disorder. And yes, there have been suicides. The perimenopause can really trigger things – women often will level out mood-wise once they are in full-blown menopause (with periods stopped for well over a year).'

According to 2019 statistics from the Samaritans,[14] the age group of women with the highest suicide rate per 100,000 in the UK is forty-five to fifty-four-year-olds (12.4 per 100,000), which is significantly higher than other age ranges. We've spoken to women who have had suicidal thoughts, and those who have come very close to actually taking their lives. The problem is very real.

> ***Tonye says:*** See your GP if you are concerned about depression and especially if you are having any thoughts about taking your life. HRT is known to work with mood in menopause. Too many women are given antidepressants rather than HRT, but they are a genuine option should you have suffered from depression before. Such approaches as CBT, mindfulness and yoga can be beneficial too.
>
> Be careful about over-the-counter medications such as St John's Wort, as it is a powerful enzyme inducer and may interact with other medications that women take. That is not to say that different supplements are not helpful, but it may be best to speak to a doctor. Diet and exercise have been found to be helpful.
>
> (Mariella says: Anecdotally, I was once prescribed St John's Wort in my twenties and it made me feel absolutely terrible, giving me palpitations and low mood at an age when I should have been on top form – so do watch out.)

Breast Changes

Did they? Did they what? Droop? Breast changes may also occur during perimenopausal years. They often become more painful before periods and more generally lumpy. Post-menopause, the tissue loses elasticity and they may therefore become less, and I mean significantly less, pert than once before. As someone who has barely ever filled a B cup, this is frustrating in one way, but at least there's not much to wave off. I've friends fortunate enough to fill larger bras, and some of them have complained that their breasts have become larger, inconvenient and – they feel – distinctly unsexy.

> ***Tonye says:*** Any lumps which concern you, get them checked. A more supportive bra might be helpful, especially if you have large breasts. Some women have mentioned an increase in cup size after starting replacement oestrogen. Sometimes, especially in women with naturally 'lumpy' breasts, this might be an issue.

Hidden Impact

Even if you don't have symptoms, your body is still going to be affected by decreasing oestrogen.

Damage caused by dwindling fertility hormones, such as loss of bone density and lack of protection from heart disease, is silent. I had a friend of my age who was lucky enough not to experience any menopausal symptoms at all, and she led an irritatingly exemplary life, eating a plant-based diet and barely drinking. She was shocked to discover at a routine health screening at fifty-eight that she had osteoporosis, and, despite her early misgivings, eventually embraced HRT, which has had a positive impact on her bone density.

'Even if a menopausal patient has no complaints, there are still health considerations that require attention,' says Professor Minkin. 'Both cardiovascular disease and bone loss are associated with the loss of oestrogen,' she advises in a 2019 article on the subject.[15] 'There are dangers from low oestrogen which aren't necessarily going to be evident for some time yet.'

It's well worth knowing that you can help yourself, and we're looking at this in more detail in further chapters.

Menstrual Migraine

This is a book about me, to an extent, but hopefully not myopically so. I have never suffered menstrual migraine (or any migraine), but have enough friends who do – and who've found them increasing in severity, frequency and duration around the menopause, with thundering pain, vomiting and days in bed in the pitch darkness – to recognize the importance of the topic.

Before asking the advice of headache specialist Professor Anne MacGregor, I did lots of research into the subject of menstrual migraine, in order to sound intelligent. Or, at least, I tried. The information available – beyond acknowledging the fact that many women suffer menstrual migraine and may suddenly develop excruciating and life-changingly debilitating headaches from their early forties onwards – simply doesn't exist.

Anne has been fighting this for over three decades. She is still trying to raise adequate funding to do the research linking migraine with hormonal changes, and fought to get menstrual migraine recognized in the classification of headache disorders.

'These are migraines which can start in your teens or twenties and may not become a problem until early to mid-forties. As women approach menopause, migraine, and particularly perimenstrual migraine, is likely to become more prevalent. Post-menopause, you start to see improvement.' As ever, it's the fluctuating hormones that are responsible.

'It's known that there are often links between oestrogen and migraine, and that they are more frequent among perimenopausal and menopausal women. Thousands of women are being left in limbo, where they can't work full time and feel isolated and depressed, but they are not being offered effective treatment.'

Because they're not continuous, they're not considered particularly disabling. Yet, says Anne, migraine has been recorded by WHO as being the leading cause of years lost to disability during women's reproductive years. 'I've spoken to women who take days off every month as annual leave, or who are doing part-time work because they don't feel they can hold down a full-time job. It can be utterly devastating, affecting relationships as well as careers, and also very frightening, even though it's effectively the brain taking a holiday from too much stimulus.'

In a recent review of the women attending her menopause clinic in London, over forty per cent of them were currently experiencing migraine. The majority of these women weren't getting adequate treatment, with only twenty per cent on migraine-specific medication. 'Most were being treated with paracetamol, which is the least effective available medication for migraine.'

The unpredictability of menopause doesn't help. 'Don't forget that oestrogen spikes as well as declines during menopause, which is bad news for those suffering from migraine,' says Anne.[16]

Anne says: While HRT has little effect on migraine post-menopause when the ovaries have become quiet and natural oestrogen levels are low and stable, HRT during perimenopause can add to daily fluctuations of the natural ovarian cycle, especially if you are taking oral HRT. Where possible, we shut down the ovarian cycle with hormones until the ovaries themselves become quiet, replacing the oestrogen as necessary. Migraine and headaches generally are affected by hormones and so can worsen around menopause. The research shows that there is a link between migraine and the severity of flushes and sweats. There is no research showing that treating flushes and sweats helps migraine but, clinically, stabilizing hormone fluctuations with HRT does benefit migraine in some women. This is why individual treatment is so important.

Can We Blame the Menopause?

Here is another problem, which flows seamlessly from the above concerns. I don't want to give the impression that all women over the age of forty are stumbling around, incoherent with exhaustion and rage, but unable to articulate their feelings because of brain fog! That's not how it manifests. Work, relationships and family will be prioritized and – usually – fulfilled. The only people punished are ourselves.

On this note, it's worth pointing out that I entirely blame my menopause for my not having had the fiftieth party to end all parties. With my anxiety levels and insomnia off the Richter scale, the thought of being responsible for a knees-up fit for five decades on the planet was way too onerous. Instead, as that auspicious birthday approached, I felt more like crawling under a shell than donning my glad rags and hitting the dance floor, as had been my intention for a decade.

In the end, I was luckily rescued from my determination to stay in with my husband and young kids (or, better still, send him out), hiding from the world, and was overridden by my friend Amy, who refused to allow me that luxury. So it passed with a properly age-appropriate surprise dinner party at the Wolseley for a tiny group of friends. When I look back on myself then, from my devil-may-care post-menopause prime, I barely recognize that shrinking violet. What a difference a few years on the right hormones can make! My fifty-fourth birthday, in contrast, was a raucous all-night party for two hundred, complete with live music.

Returning to my experience, permanent exhaustion, irritability and brain fog may feel as though they affect every single part of your life, sapping the joy, destroying self-confidence and removing the ability to perform as well as you want – whether it be at work or home – and affecting your closest relationships.

So now – in retrospect – I realize I'm one of millions who suffered from bewilderment and self-castigation, rather than swift recognition and diagnosis – which in itself can give relief. Many of my contemporaries are now enduring this – and far, far worse – in ashamed or puzzled silence. It took me two years to seek help – and I am certainly no stoic.

The unique experience

Finally, every woman's menopausal journey to the final stage of full maturity will be completely different. Where one forty-nine-year-old woman may have thirty hot flushes a day, her friend of the same age will have none.

That's why this transitional phase in our biological lives needs individual and expert assistance to navigate, even if you're one of a small minority who notice nothing at all (in which case, I suspect you're unlikely to be reading this!).

For example, the North American Menopause Society suggests that seventy-five per cent of women may have a hot flush (or hot flash, as they call the phenomenon) during perimenopause. Our very own British Menopause Society cites another study, pointing out that onset of moderate to severe hot flushes happens aged forty-five to forty-nine years, and that African-American women have a longer duration of hot flushes compared to white women. The phenomenon can last – continues the study quite blithely – between 3.84 years and more than 11.57 years.[17]

> Yet still so many of us are left to flounder in a turbulent sea of hormones without proper care or assistance for the perplexing symptoms.

That's just two studies into one single symptom. Three quarters of us may or may not suffer to some degree for an unspecified amount of time. You see the problem in trying to make any sort of generalization?

It seems obvious that attempting to deal with menopause as a universal condition to 'herd medicate' (I use the term ironically!) doesn't work. Yet still so many of us are left to flounder in a turbulent sea of hormones without proper care or assistance for the perplexing symptoms. This entirely individual experience is seldom recognized as such in either the mythology or mainstream medical practice, and diagnosis relies heavily on our ability to intuitively recognize the changes occurring in our bodies and then demand the help and medication we might need. Sadly – as many of us have found out – our own self-knowledge isn't always respected by the medical profession.

As I've already said, your mother's experience is likely to be a good starting point for your own (so, if she's still about, I can't recommend strongly enough that you try to have the conversation), otherwise there is no way of ascertaining what yours will be. If you could predict your menopause, then you could prepare for it, but, for my generation and maybe even that of my daughter, it's still an unattainable dream.

The childless impact

PSYCHOTHERAPIST, FOUNDER OF GATEWAY WOMEN
AND AUTHOR OF *LIVING THE LIFE UNEXPECTED:*
HOW TO FIND HOPE, MEANING AND A FULFILLING
FUTURE WITHOUT CHILDREN JODY DAY, FIFTIES

If, like me, you had wanted to have children, can you imagine the complexity of arriving at mid-life without them? For involuntarily childless women, the menopause is the end of any last smidgen of hope we might be harbouring. People say it's not possible to 'grieve something you've never had', but it most definitely is. It's called 'disenfranchised grief' and it's a devastating loss – even more so as it's one that most people don't let you talk about, but instead close down your pain with responses like, 'Well, you can always just adopt' (from someone who has no experience of the emotional and logistical hoop-jumping involved) or 'Kids aren't all they're cracked up to be, you know!' (from someone who never stops banging on about how #blessed she is as a mother on social media . . .).

The existential pain of childless grief at the same time as the final 'full stop' of the menopause can be so intense that I've referred to it as 'a death you survive'. It's a life-changing dark night of the soul that deserves much greater respect and sympathy than it currently receives in our grief-phobic and grief-illiterate culture.

I was forty-four-and-a-half (those halves matter during your 'still hopeful' years) when my second post-divorce relationship ended and I realized – finally – that I would never have children – that childlessness wasn't just going to be a chapter on my path to motherhood, but the whole story. The grief I felt was immense, although I didn't know it was grief at the time. Lots of us don't, and that also includes many therapists, doctors, medics and the media. This, combined with the bias and judgements against women who haven't given birth is quite staggering, and yet we're an average of one in five women in the UK and most developed countries, one in four in Ireland, Italy and Spain, and one in three in Germany, for example.

The 'childfree' are those six-to-ten per cent who have chosen not to be parents – a much lower number than their recent media rehabilitation might suggest. But I'm one of the 'childless', someone who wanted to be a parent and for whom it didn't happen. Ten per cent of us are childless due to infertility, but eighty per cent of women who arrive at mid-life without children are childless by circumstance – and those circumstances vary widely. Perhaps we didn't find a suitable or willing partner (it's called 'social infertility' and this is massively on the rise), or couldn't afford to have children, had chronic conditions which made it unwise, are recovering from trauma, or for many other (and often combined) reasons. There's a list in my book called 'Fifty Ways Not to Be a Mother', and it could easily run to one hundred.

What I didn't realize as I started my grieving process was that I was already well into perimenopause. When I missed my first period at thirty-nine, I put it down to stress (I'd recently divorced after sixteen years with my partner), and I continued to miss one period a year for the next four years. I put those down to stress, hormone problems (I thought it was my thyroid), jet lag and a fantasy pregnancy. My young female GP didn't suggest anything else, other than depression, and actually said that my realization at forty-six that my symptoms might be menopause-related was 'a brainwave'!

I knew that female fertility wound down after the age of forty, but I had no idea that this was to do with the declining quality of my eggs, nor that the process began far younger. I am saddened by how ignorant I was for a well-informed and intelligent woman, as I would have made different decisions about my 'unexplained infertility' in my marriage, had I known. And as for the 'menopause' – I just thought it meant that your periods stopped around the age of fifty-one and involved hot flushes. I had never even heard the word 'perimenopause' and was clueless about its complex and misunderstood symptoms.

When you lose your markers of fertility – strong hair, unlined skin and perhaps a small waist – people decide you are 'past your childbearing years' (just that phrase alone is so telling!), at which point you're put into a different social category as a woman. These days, we can fudge a lot of the markers of middle age with dyed hair and good dentistry. But menopause is a good reminder that we are middle-aged women, and moreover, ones who aren't respected or listened to in our culture, other than as part of the #AsAMother brigade.

There is an ancient and quite primitive unconscious prejudice against childless women which is driven by the ideology of 'pronatalism', which creates the belief that the only way to be a fully adult person is to be a parent, and that the lives and experiences of parents are more valuable than those of people without children.

This, combined with sexism, means that if you are both unpartnered by a man and childless, once you hit the menopause you are no longer part of the patriarchal project. You don't have the status of being a mother (or a potential mother), and nor do you have the protection of a man's social position. When you consider that the only positive word in the English language for an older woman is 'grandmother', you can begin to see this in action – all the popular in-use words for childless women from mid-life onwards are insults, including 'career woman', because who ever says 'career man'?!

So how do we come to terms with this and what can we do to rescue our self-worth and self-esteem from the scrapheap of society's expectations? Well, it's an inside job. We have to enter into a profound process of working out for ourselves what our value is now the dream (and protection) of the status of motherhood and grandmotherhood is closed to us. We have to root out the pronatalism that pervades our society, where it lives in our own consciousness, and stop buying into the idea that we are 'less than' mothers. We need to radically liberate ourselves from the notion that we have done something 'wrong' by being childless that we need to 'make up for'. As a society, we don't need everyone to be having children, but we do need support for those who do, and more empathy for those who are grieving that this is not the case for them. Adults without children contribute hugely and willingly to the civic society that other people's children rely upon – it's time to start seeing us as part of the human family, not as misfits. We matter too – and so does our experience of menopause.

Miscarriages marked my menopause

DESIGNER PEARL LOWE, EARLY FIFTIES

These days, every single morning, I wake up excited about the day ahead. But, for five years, at least fifty per cent of the time, and especially in the two weeks before my period, I just wanted to go back to bed as soon as I opened my eyes. I was crying, feeling down, and couldn't really cope very well generally. I wasn't a happy person. Now, post-menopause, I am happy most of the time. I take things in my stride, things bother me less and apparently I don't shout as much.

I only realized that I was entering the menopause when I

was forty-two; my husband Danny and I were trying for a fifth baby, but I kept having miscarriages. I had three in a row and the last one – devastatingly – was at five months. After that, I had hormone tests, which revealed that I was perimenopausal. 'But that's really early,' I said, horrified. The doctor reassured me that I was right at the beginning. 'I don't think you'll be able to have another baby, though.'

After this, I had five years of symptoms: very heavy bleeding and insomnia, as well as feeling so fatigued during the day, I had to go to bed in the afternoon. I was unbelievably tired. And I was horrible. Very angry, and very down. I think of those years as being not much fun and, in retrospect, I suspect that my yo-yoing hormones have always caused problems. I struggled with my mental health in my twenties and thirties, and I now wonder whether my hormones were out of sync. I certainly know that I'm happier without having the fluctuations.

Aged forty-seven, I went to see a doctor in London and she suggested HRT 'to keep your collagen and stay happy'. What a difference it made! I rub in oestrogen gel in the morning and take a micronized progesterone pill called Utrogestan in the evening, which sends me off to sleep. They gave me testosterone gel as well, but it made me feel high, and because I'm now sober (since 2005), that's not great.

It is such a relief to have everything over. It's hard to say that my even mood these days is entirely down to stable hormones, because the four kids were pretty young when I was in my thirties, so I was also exhausted. But I'm not on a yo-yo the whole time. I thought there was something wrong with me, and everything was a bit of a nightmare. Now I feel that life is bright and optimistic. Some women say that they find more drive after the menopause. I've found that having just two kids at home means I can really focus and create. I've spent thirty-one years doing the school run. I've paid my dues! I'm not driven by ambition, but the need to make things which I can't find in the shops. I've not lost my urge to nurture, but I don't want more kids anymore, and I'm not quite ready to be a grandmother. Babies aren't on my agenda in any way, even if I can pass them back.

Serena Mackesy

BEST-SELLING AUTHOR SERENA MACKESY
(AKA ALEX MARWOOD), FIFTIES

I'm divided on the menopause. I'm fully aware that I've been relatively lucky in that I've not gone through pure hell. But there's still part of me saying, 'Oh, for God's sake, it's just a thing and part of life.' You are at the mercy of your hormones all your life. Periods are such a pain in the arse: they're traumatic when you first get them – it's impossible to believe that your nice, clean body is so mucky – and then, in middle age, the awfulness of them starts to become unpredictable. Every woman has a tale of terrible blood-related humiliation, and the chances of that go up once you're perimenopausal. I unexpectedly got my period on a remote island in Thailand when I was in my early forties. You can only imagine the hell of trying to find sanitary products.

I started getting terrible hot flushes in my mid-forties. I've always been prone to overheating, but by my early fifties I'd suddenly wake up in the middle of the night with a wet bed. Or I would go bright red and have to sit down. I started taking a fan with me everywhere I went. It's interesting that you have to do your own research, because doctors don't seem to be good at connecting things.

Joking one's way through these things is bloody helpful. I remember going through Heathrow airport once, and security was very slow. I could feel myself getting worked up, and that can tip over into a hot flush. I got pulled over, and this young chap in his twenties was going through my bag, taking everything out, and by this point I was having the most enormous red, sweating hot flush. He looked up and said accusingly, 'You're sweating! Why are you sweating?' I looked straight at him. 'Because I'm a middle-aged woman, sonny.' He went scarlet and put everything away. I've certainly never been coy or apologetic, or seen any reason to be so.

I felt liberated from my periods

RETIRED MATHS TEACHER ALTHEA STEVENS, SEVENTIES

I reached menopause in my early fifties. I had hot flushes then, and I still get them now, but nothing I can't handle. I treated the whole thing as a liberation and freedom from severe period pain; from PMT, which caused real problems for me and for my marriage; from mess and discomfort; from migraines and awful mood changes.

Hallelujah! was my reaction.

I don't remember any mood issues, I never felt that my femininity was threatened and I didn't try any treatment of any kind. I just celebrated. I did gain weight very suddenly, but dealt with that by eating carefully for a while, then the weight went down and stayed that way. I didn't take HRT or anything. To be honest, I didn't need it.

I still look on that time as the best thing that had happened to me for years. For the first time since I was thirteen, I felt free from having my body drag me down.

How a hot flush feels

PROFESSOR OF SOCIAL INTERACTION AT LOUGHBOROUGH
UNIVERSITY ELIZABETH STOKOE, FORTIES

As my friends will know, I am generally freezing cold, with hands that look dead between October and May. The prospect of perimenopausal hot flushes didn't seem that bad, but FFS. They are! They come in waves every couple of hours, day and night, and during them I am drenched in sweat. But it's not just about being hot, as anyone who has experienced these things will know. So, for those of you who haven't, or won't, and want to understand your friends and partners, this is how it feels. Imagine that, with absolutely no warning, you're injected with a hefty dose of the flu virus, and simultaneously transported to a sauna with your winter coat and several blankets on. At any time. During meetings. On a stage. Over dinner. In the cinema. Sitting on the train. A few minutes later, you're fine (and, if you're me, freezing cold again!). I had hoped that the universe might throw me a bone and give me no menopause (or at least no symptoms), to make up for not being able to have kids – and there's barely any advice for women in my position. Upshot: if you see me looking like I've stepped into a shower, you'll know what's happening.

I tried to take my life

FOUNDER OF MENOPAUSE SUPPORT UK
DIANE DANZEBRINK, FIFTY-FOUR

I was only forty-five when I picked up our four beloved Jack Russells, put them in the back of the car and started to drive, as though in a trance. There's a major road near our house, and I was just seconds away from driving under an enormous lorry when one of the dogs started barking. I was brought sharply back into the moment and was horrified at just how close I'd come to ending everything. Somehow, I managed to drive home very slowly, and told my husband what had happened.

The possibility of women wishing to take their lives during menopause cannot be dismissed. At the age of forty-four, I had a total hysterectomy for suspected ovarian cancer. I was thrilled to be given the all-clear, and thought I'd just get on with life. In the six weeks after the operation, I found that I was having hot flushes, but I was so thrilled to be recovering that I was happy to put up with them. My GP briefly mentioned HRT, but I didn't want it as I had heard so many awful things, so I saw a private nutritionist and took her advice about vitamins and herbal supplements. And that, I thought, was the end of it.

But, about four months after the surgery, things started to change dramatically. I felt anxious the entire time. I was struggling to sleep and having panic attacks. I was frightened to be on my own and stopped leaving the house. I couldn't answer the phone, walk the dogs or see friends. I couldn't even open an envelope. My world was so dark that I felt as though I was existing under a black cloud the entire time. I was a husk of my former self.

After my near-death experience, I saw a doctor who was the first to explain how vital HRT was in my case. I felt better after a couple of weeks, but then I started to get angry. What about the women whose little dogs didn't bark at just the right time? The women who didn't have decent family support? I found chatroom after chatroom online, with women saying that they felt as though they were going mad. I was staggered that I wasn't given more advice following my operation, and that's what inspired me to start educating women about the menopause.

Swollen eyelids

WRITER LORRAINE FISHER, FIFTIES

It seems an odd thing to remember, but the day before Prince Harry and Meghan's wedding in 2018, aged forty-nine, I was having lunch with work colleagues and could hardly see a thing because my eyelids were so swollen. This happened every single morning for six months. When I went to Israel on a work trip, I had to wear sunglasses the entire time, and every day started with half an hour of cold compresses. It coincided with a whole raft of menopausal symptoms, which I was desperate to alleviate.

I had been refused HRT, aged forty-six, when I first went to the doctor with irregular periods and low mood. Because my dad died before he was sixty, and my brother had a heart attack at fifty-four, I was warned that the risks were too high, even though I begged. But, although they both smoked, I don't. I have good blood pressure and no diabetes. When she did blood tests and discovered that I had poor thyroid function, I was just given thyroxine.

That refusal impacted my life for three years. I was prescribed beta blockers for my low mood, which made me dizzy to the point of almost fainting on occasion. A great deal of my job was doing investigations into animal cruelty. I became incredibly anxious about being sued and got very upset about the animals. Effectively, I could no longer do my job.

Once I finally got HRT, in 2020, after seeing three doctors, I felt as though part of my life had been stolen. I was incredibly relieved. It was just before the first Covid-19 lockdown in 2020, and I had an incredibly ill dog. Imagine no HRT and a dying animal.

The Bad Rap of HRT

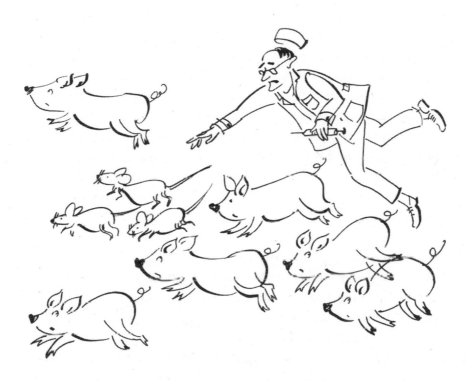

'There seems to have been quite a race to work out what was going on,
and a great number of rats and pigs dying (and, presumably, a few
female human casualties further down the line) for the cause.'

My appreciation of Hormone Replacement Therapy, or HRT, has been well broadcast. It's no exaggeration to say that it restored my quality of life at the age of fifty-one, and has contributed to maintaining my state of health, hope and (mostly) happiness ever since. There are – it's often stated – few certainties in life. But I'd add to the depressing clichés of death and taxes the absolute and cheerful knowledge that, barring true disaster, such as global shortage, I will take HRT until I turn up my toes. My tube of oestrogen gel will have to be prised from my cold hands, which will be clutching it at the moment my soul departs from my body. That's how strongly I believe in it. But, as you know, whether or not to take it is as hotly debated and more passionately argued than communism, immigration, Brexit, the right way to poach an egg, whether you have a cold or flu, and if boot-cut jeans really are back in fashion.

Many of you probably don't believe that HRT is a good idea, and it's a choice that is, and absolutely should be, up to the individual. But we can only make good decisions when we are armed with accurate information. Around HRT there remains a hotchpotch of conflicting advice. I absolutely respect anyone who doesn't wish to take it, but it's important to contextualize why we are all to this day nervous about something that has the proven potential to make you feel better. Simply put, there is still an ingrained fear that HRT might be the cause of your early death, when the evidence suggests that you are less likely to die prematurely if you are taking it.

Memories are long, especially when it comes to health scares, and dirt sticks. If you have qualms about the safety or efficacy of HRT, it is almost undoubtedly because of the lasting effects of a couple of studies back in the early Noughties, and especially a report in 2002. At this time, a project known as the Women's Health Initiative made global headlines when it claimed that oestrogen-and-progestogen-combined HRT increased the likelihood of a multitude of health problems, including the risk of breast cancer. Until this point, it had been liberally prescribed in the UK. But hundreds of thousands of women subsequently binned their prescriptions.

Many breast cancer survivors, such as the presenter Jenni Murray, whom I interviewed for my documentary about the menopause, feel strongly that HRT is a contributing factor in their developing it.

Google HRT and, to this day, thousands of websites still issue dire warnings, which are now years out of date. Thankfully, scientific opinion has shifted, and we are able to put those fears into context.[1] For most of us, the benefits far outweigh the risks, but it has taken two decades to start undoing the harmful propaganda.

Let's have a quick trot through the development of this controversial medication.

The horrible history of HRT

The development of HRT was conducted by men, whom it would benefit almost as much as the women for whom it was prescribed. Imagine the agony of living with a menopausal woman; all that flushing and forgetfulness. No man should have to suffer like that.

As far back as 1897, it was reported that ovarian extract helped with hot flushes.[2] The 'modern theory of menstruation', as described by the American/Czech gynaecologist Emil Novak in 1921, said that the ovary governs menstruation by secreting a hormone – a word which was first used in 1905 by Ernest Starling, a professor of physiology at University College London, and which comes from the Greek – meaning 'to excite'. It was a trio of men who isolated and purified oestrogen from the urine of pregnant women around 1929; Edgar Allen and Edward Adelbert Doisy worked together in the States, and German scientist Adolph Butenandt separately. Manly handshakes, back slaps and career prestige all round. Oestrogen was, quite rightly, perceived as a miracle substance.[3]

Incidentally, the word 'oestrogen', or 'estrogen', comes from the Greek. It's with a raised eyebrow and eyes rolled all the way back in my head that I impart the knowledge that *oistros* means 'mad desire' and *gennan* 'to produce'.[4] Us women, eh! Back in the day, it was no easy process procuring this precious chemical; in the 1930s, it took four tonnes of sows' ovaries to isolate 12 mg of oestradiol – a form of oestrogen. Consider that a single pump of the gel we rely on today is likely to deliver 0.75 mg of this precious ingredient. If, like me, you rely on two or three pumps daily, that's barely a week of relief, and would call for the sacrificing of many sows. Then, in 1934, crystalline progesterone was isolated from the ovaries of 50,000 pigs.

I am simplifying the story enormously. There seems to have been quite a race to work out what was going on, and a great number of rats and pigs dying (and, presumably, a few female human casualties further down the line) for the cause.[5]

The commercial development of HRT began with the production of a substance called Emmenin in the 1930s – an oestrogen product made from human-placenta extract and used for alleviating period pains.[6]

> Incidentally, the word 'oestrogen', or 'estrogen', comes from the Greek. It's with a raised eyebrow and eyes rolled all the way back in my head that I impart the knowledge that *oistros* means 'mad desire' and *gennan* 'to produce'.

Clearly, this wasn't an especially practical approach either; there is presumably a limit to how many human placentas you can lay your hands on, so it must have been a brow-sweeping moment for women and the drug companies (and the pigs) when, around the same time, oestrogen was found in the urine of pregnant mares, and this was hailed as an easy and inexpensive alternative.

In the early 1940s, the resulting drug, Premarin (from the words 'pregnant mare urine'), was marketed commercially as an oestrogen replacement in North America and Canada, though HRT wasn't available in the UK until 1965. Incidentally, it's still prescribed, but for many, that ingredient is off-putting and there are newer, safer forms.[7]

There was an ocean of difference between HRT in the States and the UK. Across the pond, the (white, middle class) reaction to Robert Wilson's *Feminine Forever* meant that, by 1975, oestrogen was the fifth most prescribed drug. It was all rather *Stepford Wives*. In the UK we were more cautious, with just three per cent of women taking it by the mid-Seventies. There was a panic when a link was discovered between HRT and endometrial cancer, but this was resolved by adding a progesterone element.[8]

The scary studies

That brings us to the latter part of the twentieth century. 'In the Eighties and Nineties, use of HRT was fairly widespread amongst women of menopausal age,' says consultant gynaecologist and chairman of the British Menopause Society, Haitham Hamoda. There was strong feminist debate as to whether HRT was ageist and sexist, but decades of clinical studies were clear on the benefits in terms of heart disease and bone health, and women taking HRT were said to enjoy a better quality of life.

Then catastrophe hit. Nothing gives a substance a bad name like a cancer association – though, on reflection, it's odd that we continue to smoke and drink in the face of very clear evidence that both have proven links. Unless you're a raw-food-munching vegan living in the wilderness, and have zero contact with twenty-first-century pollutants, chemicals, drugs, tobacco, saturated fats or alcohol, HRT isn't making it into any Top One Hundred 'Steer Clear' list.

Medics were aware of the possibility of an HRT/breast cancer link, but overall studies were positive. The news that stopped millions of women overnight was the 2002 report by the Women's Health Initiative (WHI) in America, stating that researchers had ended the combined HRT part of the study early because women taking it were more at risk of breast cancer, heart disease, stroke and blood clots.

The headline on the initial press release read: 'NHLBI Stops Trial of Estrogen Plus Progestin Due to Increased Breast Cancer Risk, Lack of Overall Benefit'.[9] Well, you wouldn't take it, would you? It seems irresponsible to eagerly consume a medicine that might kill you. The problem was that this wasn't true, and there were major concerns with how the survey was conducted and the study findings were interpreted and presented.

Fears were further compounded the following year by the 2003 Million Women Study (MWS) in the UK, which raised similar concerns. 'Here, there were significant flaws in its methodology and design which should limit the application of its conclusions,' says Haitham. The many existing positive studies were ignored. Facts, as we've come to recognize, travel an awful lot more slowly than scary news.

In 2017, one of the principal investigators in the WHI study, Robert D. Langer, MD, MPH, Professor Emeritus of Family Medicine and Public Health at the University of California, San Diego, wrote a paper explaining that, when the initial results were assessed, most of the participating investigators, including several physician-epidemiologists like himself, were excluded. In fact, before he and his colleagues could intervene and correct the paper, it had been finalized for publication.

He said then: 'That headline, pandering to women's greatest fear – the fear of breast cancer – ensured that word of the study would spread like wildfire. And it ensured that the conversation would be driven much more by emotion and politics than by science.'

I contacted Professor Langer to ask how he felt when he learned of the intention to publish the report. 'I was furious,' he says. 'In fact, at the investigators' meeting when we were provided with the initial paper, I and several of my colleagues attempted to introduce revisions. That proved impossible as we were told the paper was already in print. Then, when we were shown the press release as a further fait accompli and told that it too would not be changed, I had a shouting match with the programme director from the NIH, who was the first author of those materials.

'My primary point was that the intended headline was factually incorrect, extremely inflammatory and irresponsible. I said that, if the study was presented in that way, it would be impossible to have a rational discussion about HRT for years to come. I also pointed out that it was unethical to have submitted a paper in final draft to a journal, with named authors, including the majority of the investigators present at that meeting, who had not seen or approved it.'

Of the study itself, he says, 'There was a problem with the ages of women enrolled.' The average age of the women taking part was sixty-three, which is a good ten years beyond the menopause. 'It is now clear that the response of major organs in women's bodies to oestrogen changes as oestrogen levels decline. The fact is that maintaining levels beyond menopause with HRT is very different from reintroducing oestrogen ten years later.' In addition, many of the women were obese and half of them had smoked or were still smokers; both significant cancer risks.[10]

'The most egregious flaw was that the harms touted for breast cancer and heart disease were so slight that they did not cross a pre-specified threshold for statistical significance,' says Robert. 'In other words, it was scientifically wrong to say that there was harm.'

(The HRT they were taking was a form of the pregnant-horse-urine oestrogens [Premarin]. The vast majority of available research [both clinical trials and observational] reflects use of this form of oestrogen, Robert says. The progestogen used was medroxyprogesterone acetate, which is also still available.)

Imagine, if you will, how different the landscape would have been had Robert Langer and his colleagues been allowed to make corrections. He was absolutely correct in his predictions. Millions of women stopped taking HRT – the British Menopause Society says that numbers fell by sixty-six per cent.[11]

Those aren't simply numbers. They represent every woman who has crept up to me and asked for advice about their crippling menopausal symptoms. They're every woman who has chosen to endure hot flushes and bone deterioration, memory loss, vaginal dryness, hair loss and unfamiliar aches and pains, all because a misguided report told her what would happen if she caved in and sought hormonal support. Women have lost their jobs, their husbands and spent years on antidepressants because inaccurate conclusions were whisked to the front of a greedy global news cycle. The fallout from that report continues to influence our choices in spite of being disproven or caveated pretty much every year since. Women have been and still are misled about HRT in a way that is criminally impacting on our ability to manage mid-life.

Subsequent studies – including ones done by the WHI – have shown the clear benefits of HRT, but we've held onto the HRT = Breast Cancer equation. Funnily enough, headlines correcting the initial findings and taking a more balanced view never appeared, or at best were only to be found buried at the back of newspapers and websites. It wasn't so much fake news as flawed news. Corrections are not sexy or sensational. Headlines reading 'HRT is actually OK' didn't have the same attention-grabbing potential, so millions of women remained (and remain) convinced that HRT imperils their well-being.

'I believe that women who have gone through menopause since the WHI [report in 2002] have been harmed, and in many cases left to suffer with poorer health because of the unwarranted degree of fear stoked by the WHI,' says Robert.

'To be clear, HRT is not for every woman, and it – like any medical treatment – is not without adverse effects. The problem is that those adverse effects have been blown far out of proportion to the clinical and scientific reality. Moreover, it has led to the rise of many substitutes that have their own adverse effects, none of which are as good physiologically as oestrogen to address issues that women in this phase of life might wish to treat.

'Not all women have indications for HRT, but for those who do and who initiate within ten years of menopause, benefits are both short-term (relieving hot flushes and painful intercourse), and long-term (bone health, coronary heart disease risk reduction).

'It is time to get past the misinformation and hysteria generated by the highly irregular circumstances of the WHI [report] and stop denying potential benefits to women who have indications and may be helped,' he states. 'HRT is appropriate for symptomatic women within ten years of menopause who have no major contraindication. Good evidence from over fifty years of observational studies and clinical trials suggests that the benefits outweigh the risks for most women when started early. I remain passionately committed to restoring rational discourse on this hugely important topic.'

'That report set us back,' says Haitham. 'We had come to the conclusion that symptoms could be easily treated, should women wish. Then, all of a sudden, came this negative view of HRT, which carried on to 2015, when the NICE menopause guidance was published. This was not a new study as such, but it reviewed and presented the collective evidence on the benefits and risks of HRT. The latter approach is important, as it allows the evidence to be seen in the context of overall benefits and risks, thus allowing women to make informed decisions as to what would best meet their needs.'

The cautious comeback

Aside from the millions of women who were frightened of taking something with the power to protect them from unnecessary suffering, the further negative legacy of that WHI report was that it stifled further research. 'Products went out of production and companies were worried about developing further options because of the stigma,' says former vice president of the Royal College of Obstetricians and Gynaecologists, consultant gynaecologist Janice Rymer. Menopause is a massive industry, with thousands of consumers entering every year, but nobody is going to make drugs that women are too scared to take.

Don't forget that slamming shut the HRT door opened up all manner of opportunities. Without HRT, women's symptoms still continued, and they searched for costly and unproven solutions elsewhere (or suffered until they were through).

In 2015, the evidence-based recommendations for the National

Institute for Health and Care Excellence, or NICE, guidelines were finally reworked to include HRT.[12]

In the thick of the menopause at the time, I wrote about what a positive impact HRT had had on me, genuinely believing that the debate was over. The reaction I got from that piece, with total strangers stopping me on the street to ask whether they should take HRT, made me optimistic. But, in subsequent years . . . making my BBC programme and researching this book, it became clear that many women are still absolutely terrified of it.

In 2020, I and my co-author Alice attended a menopause seminar conducted by MPowered Women – a brilliant community of experts set up by the journalist Saska Graville and menopause expert Dr Stephanie Goodwin.[13] Situated at a five-star hotel in the New Forest, we were among a group of well-informed and well-educated women of our age. But we witnessed, with some shock, how badly prepared some of them were, how scared they were of taking HRT and, perhaps most frustratingly, how so many felt that there was some virtue in denying themselves treatment and suffering in silence.

One woman actually began her question with, 'I haven't given in to HRT yet . . .' Her reaction sums up the complicated messaging we're all receiving, and the very compelling reasons why we should be demanding better education and understanding of the medications available. It compounded my belief that we need a clear and informed code of practice in this country when it comes to menopause, and to look forensically at the mythology that has created so many erroneous assumptions. The determination to write this book was born that very night.

The brave shame in taking it

Janice Rymer remains frustrated about the scaremongering which still plagues HRT, in spite of the reworking of the NICE guidance. 'HRT is not as frightening as the headlines claim,' she says. 'It seems strange that there is this stoicism among very clever women about going through menopause cold turkey. Women are doing the dance of the desperate, and GPs and health professionals are still recommending that they stay away. It infuriates me. I've even heard of women going for breast screening and being told by the radiographer to steer clear of HRT.'

I concur. Rather like natural childbirth, it seemed to me at that seminar that women had been given the impression that suffering was their lot, and those who eschewed support, like refusing an epidural, were somehow 'better' for accepting the pain. There is no other human experience presumed to reward those who refuse the very thing that will make them feel better. (Incidentally, MPowered Women themselves are sensible and well-informed HRT advocates, and I hope many minds were changed that evening!)

> Supplementing your diminishing hormones isn't the same as bravely choosing to wear knee-length when miniskirts are in.

Among the emails I have received since expressing my interest in menopause, there are plenty from women who say things like, 'I don't want to take HRT,' or, 'I know it's not fashionable to take HRT, but it helps me,' as though it's shameful. Supplementing your diminishing hormones isn't the same as bravely choosing to wear knee-length when miniskirts are in. It should be a personal choice, based on factual evidence and available information. Absolutely no one should be telling you what to do unless they have a convincing medical reason to put you off. The problem with menopause is that it's rife with rumour, but low on tangible facts.

Acknowledging the risk

But what about the dangers of HRT? It would be irresponsible not to acknowledge these or to say that they are non-existent, but when you put them in context it's hard to see how those scare stories were ever allowed to flourish. Janice Rymer outlined the risks for my BBC show very clearly, and so I returned to her when writing this book. 'Twenty-three in every thousand women between the ages of fifty and fifty-nine will develop breast cancer over five years. When you add in women taking combined HRT, it's four extra cases.' This certainly puts things in perspective.

For those four women, that's clearly of massive significance. However, I learn that I'm more likely to develop breast cancer from excess alcohol than HRT; my past enjoyment of wine may yet creep up on me. Janice points out that drinking more than two units a day leads to five extra cases in every thousand women, which is concerning; I've enjoyed a bit more than that over the years!

The greatest contributor to the risk of breast cancer is obesity. Here, Janice says that twenty-four extra cases will be diagnosed in every thousand women – that's six times the risk factor. Even this isn't entirely straightforward; there are factors such as where you gain weight, and at what point in your life, but it's known that fat cells make oestrogen, which can make hormone-receptor-positive breast cancers develop and grow. Women who are overweight tend to have higher levels of insulin, which has links to some cancers, including breast cancer.[14]

None of this means that it's your fault if you develop cancer. They are risk factors, not predictions. Clearly there are lifestyle changes that can help lower the risks, such as cutting down on alcohol and being a healthy weight. There's certainly less point dabbing on the oestrogen gel, and more risk to your health generally, if you smoke, eat unhealthily and don't exercise. You can actively reduce cancer risk. For example, there are seven fewer cases of breast cancer per thousand for women who exercise for at least two-and-a-half hours a week. The BMS says there's little or no increased risk of breast cancer among women taking oestrogen-only HRT.

Let's also remember that there are women dying from *lack* of HRT. A study published in the *BMJ* in 2012 reported on a large group of post-menopausal women who took HRT for ten years, beginning soon after menopause. They had significantly reduced risk of mortality, heart failure and heart attack, without any increased risk of cancer, DVT or stroke. A 2013 study from Yale University estimated that, in a ten year stretch from 2002 onwards, nearly fifty thousand women may have died prematurely from not taking Hormone Replacement Therapy.[15]

Far be it for me to preach (OK, I preach); everyone needs to make their own choices, but I'm staggered by how the negative spin on HRT has prompted so many women to feel it's a support they should resist rather than investigate. And I'm infuriated that, if we take matters into our own hands, it doesn't necessarily follow that we're given what we need.

'HRT transforms women's lives. In the ideal world, almost a hundred per cent of women would take it. There are very few who won't benefit,' says Janice Rymer. 'But that's my view, and the bigger picture is that it should be a choice which is offered quite automatically, and long before women start to display or suffer from symptoms of menopause.' In reality, she says, only around twenty per cent of the women who might benefit from HRT are doing so. In some parts of the country it's as low as ten per cent.

As with so many aspects of this period of change, your opinion of what you need is as valid as anyone else's. Armed with facts, we are able to make judgements about risks versus results. The advice of a good doctor is always welcome, but the medical profession needs to have more confidence in diagnosing and understanding what's happening to our bodies. Until society catches up, we need to clue ourselves up on what's available and trust our instincts in terms of what we need. If this book can achieve anything useful, the most important change will be mandatory training in menopause for medics across the board, and access to menopause clinics for all!

I'll take it forever

NOVELIST SANDRA HOWARD, BARONESS OF HYTHE,
EIGHTIES

I have always felt far more comfortable having HRT than not.
I'm a doctor's daughter twice over and I don't believe in
scare stories; I'm rather fatalistic. I had an early menopause,
aged about forty-four or so, which was a disappointment, as
I longed to have another child. I used to plague my lovely
GP in Kent about things, and eventually he had a look at me
and said, 'You really aren't going to like this, but you will get
such pleasure from your grandchildren.' I went straight onto
HRT and am still on it. I never had any conscious symptoms,
but the HRT gave me a feeling of slight confidence that I
wouldn't dry up in all directions! One or two doctors have
tried to suggest I do without, which I did try for six months.
It might have been psychosomatic, but I feel far happier
having it. I'm generally more bright eyed, and my hair and
nails are in better condition. Right now, I'm fortunate, as they
seem very happy for me to carry on with a low dose, and I
fully intend to stay on it.

I was hurtled into early menopause

ACTRESS PATSY KENSIT, FIFTIES

When you're pregnant and you have a baby, you get the
books, and then the baby comes along and it's a blessing. I
remember, after a month, I said to Jim (Kerr, my then
husband), 'What have we done?' Nothing prepares you totally!

But nothing prepared me at all for the menopause. Aged
forty-five, I was whisked into hospital for an emergency
hysterectomy with suspected ovarian cancer. I had huge
tumours on my ovaries and had already had three operations;

they kept growing back. There was no time for anyone to explain about the aftermath. I had an emergency ultrasound at nine p.m. and was told that one tumour was pressing on my ovary and another on my bowel. I had to have them removed the next day. I walked down Harley Street in complete shock, sobbing and thinking, 'My God, half an hour ago life was one way, and now it might turn out to be another.' I'd lost both my parents to cancer when they were young, and I thought to myself that I'd never take life for granted again.

I was in the ICU for two days, and we discovered that I didn't have ovarian cancer, which was a huge relief. However, I fell instantly into full menopause.

I started to get terrible brain fog, which developed into anxiety. My job is about learning words and getting it right in two takes, and my previously photographic memory failed me. I had hot flushes, a dry mouth and couldn't sleep. Someone unhelpfully pointed out that I had developed a slight stutter, and I once found myself in the supermarket completely unaware of why I'd gone in, and I left with a cabbage and a pair of tights, which were neither eaten nor worn. I'd driven since the age of seventeen, and I couldn't drive. I honestly thought I might have dementia: my train of thought would just go, mid-conversation.

My lowest menopausal moment was also my most public. The hospital had given me HRT in the form of patches and creams, but I didn't feel it was working for me, so I was persuaded to try an HRT implant. The next day, I went on *This Morning*. I knew I was feeling terrible, and apologized; the implant had triggered a migraine, which made me so ill I was barely able to speak. In retrospect, I ought to have said that I was sick and left. But I'm a professional, and I soldier on, and my publishers would have been annoyed with me. What happened next was shocking. After stumbling through the interview, of course I was widely accused of being drunk or on drugs.

It was such a public moment, and I was devastated. I pride myself on my clarity. A few weeks later, I went back on the show to explain fully, and lots of people called in with their stories. Eventually, I said, 'Stop talking about my womb, get on with the show, and I'm off to have a hot flush!'

I ended up seeing Dr Amalia Annaradnam at the London Hormone Clinic, and went on compounded bioidentical hormones in the form of a lozenge containing oestrogen and progesterone, which work for me, and I have a testosterone cream, which gives me energy, but also a full beard, which I have to have threaded off! If things are stressful, I know that symptoms can flare up again and I have to remind myself to breathe sometimes. I frequently wake at three a.m., but these days I meditate, and it makes me feel centred. Most of the time, I feel myself again. If you don't have your health, you have nothing. I call menopause 'conscious puberty' and have set up an Instagram account to connect and celebrate. I love the idea that women will feel empowered to talk about their experiences if they read my story.

I hoped that I had an alternative

ALGARVE RESTAURANT OWNER HARRIET CAMPINA, FORTIES

I had the most horrendous health anxiety aged forty-two. My gynaecologist gave me an antidepressant, which I took for six months, put on weight, drank too much and felt fat and depressed. I didn't want to take HRT. I've done IVF twice and felt I'd had enough of putting hormones into my body.

Then I found a local expert, who gave me a tincture and herbs which I mixed in a tea every day. That managed symptoms for me. I also did something called seeding, where you follow the moon cycle to regulate your periods. Day one – which is the day of the new moon – to day fifteen, I took a teaspoon of sesame seeds, sunflower seeds and a cod liver oil supplement. The second fifteen days I took a teaspoon of flaxseed, pumpkin seeds and evening primrose oil. After sixty days, I was regular again. I felt calm, happy and very relaxed, and if I stopped taking them I felt very stressed again.

However, aged 48, my night sweats became uncontrollable and this solution stopped working. I have just started HRT in the form of an oestrogen gel and a micronized progesterone tablet. I'll try anything to stop feeling like this.

I just got on with it

GRANDMOTHER-OF-FOUR ROSE EAMES, SIXTIES

I was working in a laundry when I started having symptoms in my early fifties: hot flushes, which started off just in my head and neck, but over the years ended up making my entire body damp, and I had night sweats every single night. Then my periods stopped aged fifty-six and these all got worse, although they're starting to tail off a bit now. So I'd be up every night, two or three times sometimes, and soaking wet, and then go and do a job where I was on my feet for eight or nine hours a day. It was a hard job, and, looking back, I was tired for a lot of the time. We used to laugh and joke about it: I'd have a hot flush and dash outside for a few minutes, then just come in and get on with it. I'd never take HRT – I always said that was one thing I wouldn't do, but I've taken evening primrose oil for years.

I'll take the HRT when I need it

EXECUTIVE COACH AND EQUALITY TRAINER MARY DOYLE, FORTIES

Given that we disabled women are often thought of as non-sexual or non-parents, in the eyes of the general (or uninformed) public, the menopause doesn't signify the end of my womanhood, as I was not considered a sexual being to begin with. I've been very fortunate in my sexual-health life that I have not endured many of the common gynaecological problems of my peers, so I am not too daunted by the menopause ahead of me, and ignorance is bliss to me, as I have few deep insights.

I know that the public perception of disabled people as non-sexual is total BS, of course, and I have happily avoided getting knocked up my entire adult life; I didn't want to push a bowling ball out with my unique hips, or divert from my career.

Looking at the symptoms, I see that I can expect to be a bit sweaty, moody and anxious, but I'm always like that, and they're not life-changing so far. I have said to myself and my partner in recent years that my menopause will start on a Friday, I'll have a crappy weekend, maybe be a bit snappy, and it will be all over by Monday morning. I believe it will happen like this, and, if not, I'll tell the menopause to go f@@k itself, and I'll have HRT, as highly recommended by several girlfriends.

HRT Love Song

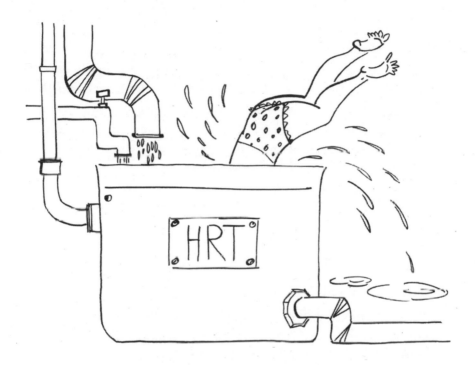

*'. . . when you're going through a catastrophic loss of hormones,
it seems sensible enough to try to top them up.'*

There is no cure for menopause, because menopause is not a 'disease', and whatever solutions you choose will simply mitigate to a greater or lesser degree the impact it has on you. But when you're going through a catastrophic loss of hormones, it seems sensible enough to try to top them up.

There are women who swear by HRT, women who swear never to take it and many others who simply don't know what to do. To add to the confusion, GPs are similarly divided, though I have to say that every single menopause expert to whom we spoke (bearing in mind they have specific and specialized training in women's health) was absolutely committed to its positive effects. Every single one.

However, not one of them recommended eye of newt and toe of frog boiled up in a cauldron at midnight and ingested by the light of a harvest moon, nor any of the extraordinary, unproven and staggeringly overpriced 'remedies' available on the internet. HRT – and I've acknowledged there are risks – has at least got countless studies proving its efficacy.

In 2014, following two years of enduring my own undiagnosed and exhausting symptoms, I was finally prescribed the first version of the non-alcoholic cocktail on which I now thrive: transdermal (absorbed through the skin) oestrogen (initially in the form of patches, which I didn't like, as they failed to break through the barrier of my body lotion); micronized progesterone, in the form of a tablet; and, initially, testosterone gel. Perhaps not overnight, but over a matter of weeks, the agonies of insomnia and the misery of being perpetually worried had faded to the back corridors of my memory. I was, to all intents and purposes, my old self, and I welcomed her. She had been absent for a long time.

I suppose I may be a bit too gung-ho when it comes to medication, as a misspent youth means that there are few drugs I haven't tried or cocktails I've turned down. Obviously, I'm not advocating a party lifestyle. One of the pleasurable aspects of speaking to a more mature (I assume) audience is a sense of diminished personal responsibility. We all know that bending over a loo seat with a borrowed tenner, a bag of (mostly) baking powder and a new best friend isn't a good look at any age, but definitely not post-fifty. If you don't know what I'm talking about, then I applaud your sensible life choices.

That cautionary note aside, middle age is surely no time to turn down substances that genuinely improve your quality of life. In truth, after two years of debilitating symptoms, I'd have probably embraced heroin if someone had told me it would help, but luckily I wasn't mixing in such circles.

When my gynaecologist first suggested I try HRT – predominantly to preserve bone density as I edged towards osteoporosis, but also to help with my poor sleep and anxiety – I was only too happy to slap on a patch and bugger the consequences. At that point, like most women, I thought I knew about the risk HRT might pose when it came to breast cancer, but it seemed worth taking it for the sake of a good night's sleep, the end of early-hours anxieties, a boost to my bone and heart health, as well as possibly lowering of the chance of type 2 diabetes and – potentially – Alzheimer's disease. I was wary, having suffered from lumps in my breasts (benign and transitory) in the past. I now have a regular breast check.

But I have heard countless stories about women being refused HRT. It's amazing how many opinions there are about what women should and shouldn't do with our bodies, and how much pain we ought to endure . . . that don't come from women themselves. As delivery vessels for the species, we've been considered common property since time began. Decisions about what is and isn't best for us have, for thousands of years, been made by people with an entirely different perspective, plus a penis.

We now understand that the physiological differences between men and women are far more extensive than simply having different sex organs. The fact that women are governed by oestrogen and men by testosterone means that our reactions to many conditions are different. But how can men possibly comprehend specifically female experiences, such as childbirth, pregnancy, periods and menopause, let alone the need to alleviate them?

A friend of mine explains the lack of male empathy for female complaints (clearly, this is a massive generalization) by pointing out that her husband was dismissive to the point of rudeness about the agony of childbirth, but incredibly loving whenever she had a hangover. 'He understood that pain, so he was able to empathize,' she says (incidentally, they are now divorced).

I'm pretty sure that almost every woman of menopause age, regardless of symptoms, has a strong opinion about HRT, and most middle-aged men don't. One woman recently told me that her GP stated that he didn't 'rate' HRT, so wasn't going to prescribe it for her. She could apparently do perfectly well without it. I wonder what study his opinion was based on, or whether he'd just been flicking through his morning newspaper . . . or whether he ever posed himself the same question before taking a painkiller or Viagra?

> It's amazing how many opinions there are about what women should and shouldn't do with our bodies, and how much pain we ought to endure . . . that don't come from women themselves.

What is HRT?

'HRT, or Hormone Replacement Therapy, is quite simple,' says Janice Rymer, Professor of Gynaecology at King's College London School of

Medicine and former vice-president of the Royal College of Obstetricians and Gynaecologists. 'When those egg-ripening follicles start to decrease in number and the body can't produce sufficient oestrogen, it all goes belly up. HRT replaces the three key hormones made by the ovaries: oestrogen, which affects every organ in the body, progesterone and – if necessary – testosterone. Short term, HRT can relieve such symptoms as night sweats, anxiety, brain fog, sleep problems and hot flushes. Long term, it protects against heart disease, certain cancers and osteoporosis.'

What type should you have? The HRT 101

While I do occasionally look back to my first, mostly medication-free, four decades, my current reliance on a daily squirt of gel and nightly popping of a pill seems a small price to pay for so many health benefits. It took a few months to find the right cocktail, but it really works for me. As every woman's menopause is different, so you are entitled to a personalized prescription. What suits one woman may be catastrophic for another. There are more than fifty variations available: patches, pills, gels and even implants. How on earth do you know which one you should take?

Dr Tonye Wokoma says:
The best formulation is the one that is right for you, and depends on your medical background and family history. There is no one-size-fits-all. If you try one and it doesn't work, speak to your GP or menopause clinic.

If you still have a womb (i.e. you haven't had a hysterectomy), you need combined HRT, where you take oestrogen and a progestogen – either micronized progesterone or a synthetic progestogen. (This word is used as the generic term for this group of hormones, with progesterone being the main one in the human body.) This is needed to keep the lining of the womb thin and healthy. Without progestogen there is a small increased risk of womb cancer. If you don't have a womb, you will probably be prescribed oestrogen-only HRT.

There are two types of combined HRT. Firstly, there's sequential or cyclical HRT, which is used in perimenopause, where you have a regular withdrawal bleed. Alternatively, the Mirena Intrauterine System (IUS) is licensed to protect the womb lining. This delivers progestogen to the womb, with the added bonus of protecting against pregnancy. It consists of a T-shaped piece of plastic, which is inserted into the womb and has two thin threads hanging through the cervix. Obviously, you have to have it inserted, which can be a bit uncomfortable, but once in it lasts five years. Lots of women don't have any bleeding with it, and you can take daily oestrogen in your preferred form.

Secondly, there's continuous combined HRT, which is appropriate for post-menopause. Here, you take oestrogen and a progestogen every day and you don't have a bleed.

HRT comes as various preparations: tablets, patches, gels, sprays and – rarely – implants. You can – in the case of gel and patches – tailor the dose to your needs; one or two squirts of oestrogen gel rubbed into the inner thigh daily is generally enough (but sometimes more is needed).

The benefit of transdermal (absorbed through the skin) HRT is that there is no increased risk of blood clots. If you take tablets, there is a small risk. But some women prefer the ease of tablets.

Hard to know, you'll be thinking, when you can change from cyclical to continuous combined. The rule of thumb for changing is to swap at the age of fifty-five, as most women would be post-menopausal by then. However, if a woman starts a sequential preparation about nine months after her last period, it is likely that she would be post-menopausal one to two years later, and she does not need to wait till she is fifty-five.

Incidentally, many women are progestogen sensitive. If you had PMS when younger, then you may find that this is the case, and an alternative regime may be to take micronized progesterone (which comes as a separate pill) for two weeks out of every twelve, rather than two weeks in four. (This is where the Mirena IUS comes in handy as well.)

If you have irregular bleeding on HRT, it may settle down

(hopefully the case if taking a synthetic progestogen in a combined preparation), but you may need a bit more micronized progesterone, or you can use a Mirena IUS. If it doesn't stop it needs investigation. Micronized progesterone can also have a sedative effect, and Mariella takes it daily to help sleep.

Another option for post-menopause is a tablet called tibolone, which is slightly different. It's a sex steroid and works on receptors in the body to make oestrogen, progesterone and testosterone.

A significant number of women benefit from the addition of testosterone. The ovaries continue to make it after the menopause, but levels will drop. Low testosterone can mean tiredness, lack of energy and reduced libido. Try oestrogen-based HRT first; this may be sufficient for managing symptoms. It is likely, incidentally, that a testosterone prescription would be initiated by a menopause specialist rather than your GP, but this may be different in different areas.

Menopause care is an art, involving evidence-based medicine, good communication and interpersonal relationships with patients, identifying and meeting them at their point of need and supporting them along this journey. There are so many permutations. Every woman is different and this needs to be recognized.[1]

Bioidentical/body identical

The most recent types of HRT are known as body identical. With the same molecular structure as the hormones that we produce in our bodies, they have fewer side effects and risks. Available on the NHS and privately, the oestrogen (as estradiol) is in the form of patches or gel. The progestogen is micronized progesterone made from yams, and available as a tablet. They are often considered the gold-standard option. In fact, a 2018 systematic review revealed that taking micronized progesterone doesn't increase the risk of breast cancer within five years, and there is 'limited evidence' that there's an increased risk after five years. This is promising news.[2]

Body identical HRT is also known as regulated bioidentical

hormone replacement therapy (rBHRT) and is different from compounded bioidentical hormone replacement therapy (cBHRT), which takes the form of personalized prescriptions offered in the private sector.

Official bodies cannot recommend compounded bioidentical hormones, as they haven't been subjected to the same rigorous testing and trials as the regulated products. 'There is no consistency with the ingredients or doses, and the people promoting them often charge women a lot of money for unnecessary, expensive tests,' says Janice Rymer.

Vaginal oestrogen

We cover dry vaginas, so to speak, in chapter ten (see page 235), but it's worth mentioning vaginal, or local, oestrogen here. This has no cancer risk at all, and there are plenty of new preparations – pessaries, gel, tablets and creams that are applied locally and are beneficial for the vagina and the bladder – both of which rely on oestrogen to stay supple and lubricated. By the way, you can have HRT and vaginal oestrogen at the same time.

There are huge benefits from making HRT your first rather than last port of call, and a vast body of evidence suggesting that, if you want the most out of it and you want it to be as safe as possible, then don't think of it as the last resort. It's proven and it's an almost-free (on the NHS) solution, which may solve many of your problems.

One of the most frequently asked questions is how long you can take HRT for. Tonye says that the NICE (official) guidance isn't entirely prescriptive or dogmatic. 'Many women are under the impression that it ought to be consumed in low quantities for as little time as possible. This is not true. NICE recommends a menopause review on an annual basis, and looking at risks weighed against benefits. My feeling, and that of many fellow experts, is that, yes, it's medication, but you should be allowed to take it for as long as you need to. This may mean as long as you live, ideally starting within ten years of the menopause or before you reach the age of sixty. This is what's known as the window of opportunity for cardiovascular benefit for HRT. The benefits outweigh the risks.' She adds that it can be started post sixty.

Women are very bad at looking after themselves, probably because we spend so much time looking after everyone else. When it comes to mid-life, it's no longer a choice; it's essential that you take the time for self-care.

Protect the heart

There's a duo of body parts that are very much supported by HRT. The heart and bones both concern me in a personal way.

Heart and circulatory diseases are the biggest killers of women in the UK. Women are far more likely to develop coronary heart disease once we lose the protection of oestrogen, and it is a condition which kills more than twice as many women as breast cancer. This is a state of affairs only recently recognized and promoted to the general public. According to the British Heart Foundation, there are around 3.6 million women living with a heart or circulatory disease (including coronary heart disease and stroke), and around twenty-four thousand women a year die from coronary heart disease in the UK – that's sixty-five women per day.[3]

'We know that before the menopause women have a far lower incidence of coronary heart disease than men,' says Barbara Kobson, senior cardiac nurse at the British Heart Foundation. 'As soon as they hit menopause and their oestrogen drops, they start to have the same risk.'

The reason for this is that oestrogen helps to control cholesterol levels and reduces the build-up of plaque which narrows the arteries in a condition known as atherosclerosis. Once oestrogen goes down, there's a higher risk of this plaque building up, so you are more likely to develop coronary heart disease or suffer a stroke.

Fluctuations in hormones during the menopause may also lead to palpitations, which can be uncomfortable. Tonye says that, if you take HRT within that aforementioned 'window of opportunity' (see page 106), then there are protective benefits for the heart. 'The plaque, or atherosclerosis, won't have had time to form in the arteries, which is what starts to happen without the benefits of protective oestrogen.' The British Menopause Society concurs.

In a double whammy of injustice, women fare far worse in the event of a heart attack. Most clinical studies have considered the male physique. Indeed, for many years, misdiagnosis of women's heart disease has been one of the shameful failures of the medical profession. In 2019, the British Heart Foundation produced a briefing called *Bias and Biology* about how the gender gap in heart disease may be causing women to die unnecessarily: a woman is fifty per cent more likely than a man to receive the wrong initial diagnosis for a heart attack.

Not all people having a heart attack get central crushing chest pain, although symptoms are similar for men and women. 'Women may not think that a discomfort or tightening around the chest, or jaw pain, could be the sign of a heart attack,' Barbara says. 'This means that they are presenting to hospital much later. Even when they reach hospital, doctors may not assume women are presenting with a heart attack, therefore reducing their chances of timely treatment.'

Boning up on the facts

Those at risk of osteoporosis should also consider the benefits of HRT. There is a strong inherited risk: if your mother has osteoporosis, so might you. As oestrogen goes down, so does your bone density and flexibility. Oestrogen protects osteoblasts, which are the cells that produce bone. When oestrogen levels drop, these aren't able to function effectively. In the five to seven years after menopause, when oestrogen production has plummeted, you can lose as much as twenty per cent of your bone mass, so you are more likely to suffer fractures.

HRT can be prescribed as a treatment for osteoporosis, to help stop bone loss and prevent fracture, and the British Menopause Society says that oestrogen is the treatment of choice for osteoporosis prevention in menopausal women. I was surprised to be asked to be tested for bone density before I went onto HRT and even more so to discover I was severely osteopenic. This is the stage where bones are thinning, and can lead to full-blown osteoporosis. I started taking HRT and exercising, and within two years my condition was reversed.[4]

No brainer?

Dementia is a very real and personal fear for me. My grandmother suffered from it, my mother now has it so badly she is in a care home, and her brother, my uncle, is also deep in its grip. As it is believed to travel down the maternal line, it's a concern for me and also for my children. 'Brain fog' affects many of us at this point in our lives, and HRT can help with this, but it is also thought that oestrogen is a protective factor against developing Alzheimer's. Might HRT help prevent this condition?

I read one of the most successful dementia books of 2020 with great interest. *The XX Brain* by Dr Lisa Mosconi[5] is all about preventing dementia. She says that, for women over the age of sixty, the risk of developing Alzheimer's is twice that of getting breast cancer, and investigates the possibility that taking HRT might offer some protection against dementia. To be honest, it doesn't seem to be conclusive just yet, which is disappointing.

She points out that a collation of more than eighteen studies showed that younger women (aged fifty to fifty-nine) taking HRT were thirty to forty-four per cent less likely to develop Alzheimer's. But the Women's Health Initiative Memory Study – a spin-off group from the Women's Health Initiative – looked at women older than sixty-five, and in the combined therapy group there was a doubling of dementia risk. Mosconi suggests that it appears taking HRT early, within five years of menopause, may have protective value, and many experts are convinced of benefits, but more research is clearly needed.

Reading the Alzheimer's Society website brings me to the same conclusion. Whether the oestrogen in HRT can protect the brain in the same way as it protects the heart and bones definitely needs further investigation.[6]

When HRT is a must: premature ovarian insufficiency

Premature Ovarian Insufficiency (POI) means that the menopause comes early. It can be devastating psychologically and physically. One in every hundred women under the age of forty, one in a thousand women under thirty and one in ten thousand under twenty experience POI. It can be natural or it might be as a result of surgery or cancer treatment.

Simply put, this is where the ovaries aren't working properly and stop producing eggs, years, and in some cases even decades, before they should – or they are surgically removed, which of course means that your body can no longer make sufficient oestrogen, progesterone or testosterone. Whether your POI is natural or surgical, you absolutely need HRT to protect your heart and bones up to at least the age of fifty-one.

Daisy Network is the only registered charity supporting women with POI but, they tell me, as with many things to do with women's fertility, there's a postcode lottery. Their long-term goal is to increase GP awareness so that there's a set protocol.[7]

At the moment, some women with POI are sent to endocrinologists, some to gynaecologists and some to GPs. Lack of appropriate advice can mean catastrophic health problems developing in later life. Similarly, faster diagnosis means more options in terms of having children – you may still have viable eggs, but once really bad symptoms start, it can be too late. Ovaries (if still present) don't always entirely fail, so up to five per cent of women with POI may ovulate, which can result in pregnancy.

'There can sometimes be a lack of advice given to women who have surgical menopause, where the ovaries are removed, or have cancer treatment which puts the body into menopause,' says Dr Tonye Wokoma. 'Although specialists are excellent in their specific fields, they may not be aware of the importance of menopause support.'

Conclusion

What's clear from the growing body of evidence that is finally being amassed is that some form of HRT is a vital treatment for most women. Maintaining optimal hormone levels isn't a luxury; in an ideal world, it's a necessity to keep you fit and strong for the years ahead. The longer you are without oestrogen, the more likely you are to suffer from all the other conditions I've described. If you see a GP who 'doesn't rate HRT', please insist on a second opinion.

> The longer you are without oestrogen, the more likely you are to suffer from all the other conditions I've described. If you see a GP who 'doesn't rate HRT', please insist on a second opinion.

There are plenty of alternative treatments available (many of which I cover in subsequent chapters) should you not be able to take HRT or because you don't wish to, and because it doesn't necessarily ease all symptoms.

Looking after your health in middle age, for far too many women, is a lottery dependent on where you live, what you can afford, the culture you come from and which GP you happen to see. In a modern, advanced, civilized nation, this is not an acceptable state of affairs. It's high time that a universal standard and code of practice was applied to what we can take, how we should take it and what sort of support we can expect from the NHS.

Donna Reddy

HR PROFESSIONAL DONNA REDDY, LATE THIRTIES

I don't blame anyone for my experience, but I'll do anything to raise awareness of premature ovarian insufficiency after a ten-year-long nightmare.

I only found out that I had POI because I chased up our doctor's receptionist for blood-test results in 2020. 'Oh yes,' she said. 'You're menopausal.' Then there was total silence on the line. I was so shocked and stunned, I could barely ask when I needed to come back. 'Well, you'll have to make an appointment, of course,' she said, a bit sternly. When I was finally squeezed in, a week later, the male doctor confirmed the results in a very matter-of-fact fashion. 'You aren't that young for it,' he said. There was a very strong implication that, at thirty-eight, I was pretty much past it for kids anyway. 'There's nothing more we can do,' he said dismissively. I went to the shop, bought a bottle of wine and lay on my sofa, crying my eyes out.

I'd had the contraceptive implant Implanon for years, and came off it aged twenty-nine, after which my periods were regular. But I felt there was something not quite right. I had what I thought was social anxiety and panic attacks; I felt anxious, very hot and had palpitations. Of course, now I realize that they were hot flushes. Looking back, in fact, there were so many clues as to what was happening. At that time, I was sent for an ultrasound, where the consultant realized that there was no sign of ovulation, but then I had a really heavy period, and was told that my blood tests were fine. Eventually, aged thirty-five, I lost my mother, and then my periods stopped completely. I started to have such serious anxiety that I couldn't go for lunch with work colleagues, and I was given beta blockers by my GP.

It was a nurse who realized what was happening. My copper coil didn't feel right and I was in agony. When I finally saw a nurse, she said that it had fallen out – which is almost unheard of. 'When was your last period?' she asked. 'Two years ago,' I replied. For the first time, six years after my symptoms started, the menopause was mentioned. She said she thought I might have started.

I have osteoporosis – I broke my ankle a few months after the POI diagnosis – as well as serious gum disease and bone loss. I am too old for free donor IVF, so I may not be able to have children. I finally saw a menopause doctor through the charity Daisy Network and was then put on HRT, which changed my life. I've also incorporated regular spiritual practice and alternative therapies, which have been just as significant a part of my journey from being a shell of myself to leading a happy and fulfilling life.

My oestrogen was too high

WRITER FLIC EVERETT, FIFTIES

Aged forty-six, I started waking up in the night drenched in sweat (nice). It happened about once a fortnight, and seemingly had nothing to do with having the heating on or off. It started around my sternum, weirdly, and I'd wake up, change my nightie and go back to bed. I've always had quite bad PMS, but, over the last couple of years, it has been full-on lunacy, occurring for about a week mid-cycle, and then a few days just before my period (which are still regular).

I cry, I feel hopeless despair, I truly believe nothing good will ever happen again, we're all doomed and the world is ending. Sometimes, I find my partner astonishingly irritating and yell at him because he's running the tap very loudly, or paying more attention to the dogs than me. It's derangement, pure and simple. I noticed it was beginning to be accompanied with a lovely undertow of wild anxiety, too. And insomnia; when I found myself awake at three a.m.

eating a giant bag of Walker's Thai Chilli Sensations and sobbing, I thought I might need to do something about it.

I called the GP, but you can't ask for a female doctor any more; it's a 'hub', so you get who you're given. I was given the arrogant, young male GP who knows as much about perimenopause as I do about racing bikes. He told me I should have a Mirena coil. I'm quite sensitive to medication, and I didn't want something I couldn't stop if it didn't suit me (or not without an unpleasant faff, anyway), and he was quite irritable and basically told me I was being silly, but said, 'You can see the nurse, if you want to.' Yeah, I did.

So, the nurse was great. There were no patches available, so she suggested a combination of oestrogen gel and progesterone pills. When I started on that, the PMS eased dramatically after a couple of months – it's now down to a few days of depression, rather than two weeks of total lunacy. But, I started to feel more down than I wanted to.

Luckily, I recently spoke to Dr Jan Toledano, at the London Hormone Clinic, and she was utterly brilliant. She said, if you're still having regular periods, you don't need oestrogen, and I basically had too much oestrogen in my system and should just take the progesterone. So I have been doing that, and feel much better. I think *every* woman should see a specialist menopause consultant, they should be trained on the NHS, and it should be taken bloody seriously from early forties onwards. If men had the menopause, there'd be cutting-edge research centres in every village.

I was told to come off HRT in my sixties

RETIREE JANE SMITH, SIXTY-EIGHT

I had awful problems leading up to menopause, terrible flooding, and was determined to go on HRT. I had previously read an article by Maureen Lipman saying it was the best thing she'd ever done. They don't tell you that your libido goes as well, and she mentioned one with testosterone in it. I already had one failed marriage. I didn't want another!

So, I was in my early fifties when I started, and it was wonderful. But you have to get a new prescription every year. In August 2019, I saw a terribly young doctor who said I had to come off it because I'd been taking it for far too long. I told her that my mother had been on it until she was seventy, and she always said that, when she stopped, all her bones just crumbled and fell apart.

I had terrible hot flushes almost immediately, and then around Christmas my fingers started to swell up. I had to take my rings off, and we didn't know what was going on.

The GP did various blood tests and my results came back with slightly raised liver function, which was rather alarming, so I stopped drinking alcohol. I then developed carpal tunnel syndrome. I remembered my daughter having carpal tunnel syndrome when she was pregnant, and then I remembered reading something about links between alcohol in older women and hormones. I realized that the whole thing seemed to come down to just that – hormones. So I went to a different doctor, an older woman. She agreed to give me a prescription, provided I promised faithfully to check my breasts regularly, and eleven months later my rings are back on my fingers! I've a friend whose mother finally came off it at eighty-six. I can't see that I'll ever give up.

Jane Anne James

NHS WORKER JANE ANNE JAMES, FIFTIES

I'm not medically trained, but I'm passionate about education around HRT. Running an online Facebook support group (Menopause & HRT Discussion Group), I am constantly horrified by the fact that women have no idea what they might take or why. Or the fact that what works for one doesn't work for others.

I had an ovary removed when I was forty-six because I had cysts. At the time, I was on antidepressants and had to increase the dose as I didn't feel right for two years. By forty-nine, I felt terrible: very low, snappy and I was sweating buckets. (My husband called me Meno Mary.) I started doing some research, and eventually, aged fifty, the GP prescribed Evorel Conti combined patches. But they weren't available – remember there are often inexplicable shortages of HRT – so they gave me combined tablets instead and I had terrible side effects, with spots on my boobs and swelling under my armpits. The next tablets I tried gave me such bad anxiety that I was off work for two weeks. Eventually, I accessed the Evorel Conti, and then had to go through the entire thing all over again to get testosterone for my muscle and joint pain, which the GP wouldn't give me and I finally obtained through a specialist. The confusion is staggering. I have women messaging me day and night, asking about different types of HRT, or having been given it and not knowing how to use it or where to put it. We need consolidation!

I've been on it for more than twenty years

MODEL JILLY JOHNSON, SIXTIES

I'd had problems with my nuts and bolts since the age of twenty-one, when I had my daughter Lucy. Then, aged forty-six, I couldn't sleep, I had rivers of sweat overnight and I was panting and puffed out the whole time. I felt like one of my Great Danes: my tongue was always hanging out and I was drooling and slobbering. Eventually, I had three-week periods and then one week off. At the same time, I was going to and from my osteopath with the most terrible back ache, which I never associated with my nuts and bolts.

Eventually, they decided to do a hysterectomy, or a hysterical, as I thought of it.

It was only afterwards that I realized how awful I'd felt for years. It turned out that I had such severe pelvic inflammatory disease, my uterus was tugging and pulling on my tubes.

The relief was immeasurable. I'd felt shit for years. I felt lighter, and different, as though I'd been carrying something poisoned inside me for years. The whole thing was just utterly toxic. It was as though I'd been fighting a battle with lead weights around my ankles.

When the surgeon came to see me the day after, he said, 'You don't need to worry about a thing. We've popped a pellet in, so you won't go through the menopause.' It was an oestrogen and testosterone implant, which was inserted into a little incision in my stomach – a little cocktail of hormones. Honestly, I was in my prime, and felt amazing. Every six months or so, I start to slow down and get a bit tired, as though my battery has run out. My husband Ashley notices – I stop sleeping well too. I feel like a junkie going into withdrawal. It's not the nicest, and I'm a bit like a patchwork quilt, as they have to do a new hole every time. But I don't do bikini modelling any more, so it doesn't matter! There's no way I'd ever stop it.

HRT isn't a magic bullet

DENTIST DR UCHENNA OKOYE, FIFTIES

If men got the menopause, hot flushes would be graded, like storms or earthquakes. 'It's a level-nine sweat today. I'm going to need a cold shower and a day off.' There would also, I suspect, be menopause screening at the age of forty.

As it is, I'm a female, university-educated doctor, with two masters' degrees and a business to run. Yet all I knew about the menopause was that it happened to old women and made them sweat a lot. I remember my grandma putting tissues under her armpits!

So, when I started to have symptoms at the age of forty-seven, I genuinely thought I had cancer. I've always survived on four or five hours of sleep a night, and suddenly I needed fourteen or fifteen. I had the worst brain fog and desperate muscle pain, which I now know was down to lack of oestrogen. I was pretty sure that I had ovarian cancer, as I had all the markers – my GP sent me for all the scans and mammograms to rule it out, and I was on antidepressants for my incessant crying. Eventually, a beauty-editor friend realized what was going on, and I took myself off to a private clinic, where I started HRT in the form of compounded bioidentical hormones. After eight weeks, I felt no different, and went to a different clinic. I finally ended up with the right dose and the right, body identical, medication for me.

I'll carry on taking it as long as I can, but it's not a cure-all. It's important to realize that you don't necessarily take HRT and instantly feel amazing. I am very reactive to medication, as I'm sure is the case with many women, so the balance needs to be just right. A year later, I'm still fanning myself and feeling up and down. I'm confident that I'll emerge from this, but I assumed that, once I knew what was going on, I'd take a pill which would fix me. It's not that straightforward. You need to try a few HRT combinations to find the right one.

Chemo, cancer and menopause

ADMISSIONS OFFICER JACKIE TRUELOVE,
FIFTIES

Menopause is the last thing on your mind when there's a cancer diagnosis. I know that in many ways I was fortunate. At the age of forty-nine, I had an early breast-cancer scan as part of a trial, and it was discovered that I had stage-two cancer very deep in my left breast. I'd never have seen a lump and wouldn't have gone for a scan for a couple of years. It might have been a very different outcome.

Chemotherapy was initially like that sixteen-week stage of morning sickness, where you feel grotty and wiped out. Then, after the first three lots – I had seven in total – they changed the formula and I felt utterly horrible. It was brutal and agonizing.

Menopause was a sort of side effect, in some ways. I was told that the treatment would probably make me enter it, but there are no definites. We were trying to get oestrogen out of my body, as that's what fed my cancer, so HRT wasn't an option. Sex drive wasn't exactly a priority, and neither was counting periods. Once I started taking tamoxifen, which puts you straight into menopause, I started to have hot flushes sweeping up my entire body. Compared to chemo, these are a walk in the park, but psychologically it's been challenging. I felt unfeminine and horrible, and realized I wasn't young anymore.

What's frustrating is that the menopause was an afterthought to curing the cancer, but I'm still going through it five years later, so it's hardly insignificant. My oncologist and surgeon were brilliant, but they were men, so I'm not sure they understood. Once they've done their treatment and their job, it's not their scope or problem. I actually think you need advice about it at the time and to know whether you have options.

CHAPTER FIVE

(Meno) Pause for Thought:
Breathe Deep and Find Your Tribe

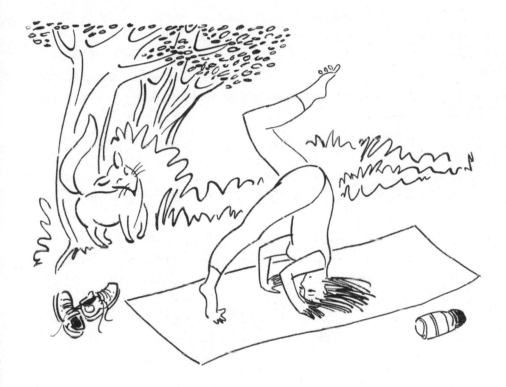

'Yoga is my other weapon against post-menopause
insomnia, stress and generally seizing up.'

Let's take a moment.

If I start chanting *Om Shanti Om*, cynics may start thinking I've finally lost my marbles. But when the going gets tough, those in the know take a few slow breaths and look deep inside for strength and awareness.[1] The link between mind and body is absolutely recognized by science, as is the fact that, if you look after either one, the other responds positively. It's a relationship we forget at our peril. That's why many women struggling with the menopause find that proven practices such as yoga, mindfulness and meditation can come in very handy indeed.

The idea that you can inhale your way through menopause is one I initially approached with cynicism. It plays to every stereotype of the hysterical woman, as well as that ill-founded philosophy purported by the likes of Freud: that women are nothing but unhinged weaklings, dominated by our inferior biology.

Nevertheless, a simple breathing technique to quieten the all-night-long chorus in my brain is one of the most helpful tools I've embraced. I've regularly lain awake in the small hours, breathing deep into my abdomen and counting each breath until my frenzied thoughts subside. There are occasions when it takes so long I lose confidence that I will find respite, but eighty per cent of the time it works. When it comes to what I term 'raging brain syndrome', a particular issue for those of us with insomniac tendencies, this is top of my list for helping shrug off negative thoughts and shepherd my meandering mind back to stillness.

Calming yourself down may sound horribly head-patting, but if you generally think of menopause as being unpleasant, or feel stressed about symptoms such as hot flushes, then it will probably have more of a negative impact. That's why the music in horror films starts putting you on edge long before the gory bits begin.

Jaws without the dum-dum, dum-dum is just a woman swimming, and *The Omen* is a kid with a grumpy face and a serious case of stink eye. Anticipation is everything when it comes to bad news stories, and this becomes a cycle of stress. The more worried you are, the more you become trapped in a sort of increasingly dark cave of negative emotion.

'Anxiety makes the adrenal gland release the stress hormone cortisol, and this fight-or-flight hormone courses around your bloodstream, pushing up your blood pressure and heart rate,' says psychologist Dr Meg Arroll. 'Long term, this impacts on our general health and immune systems.' But, she points out, we can choose to alter our thoughts and therefore control our cortisol levels. Effectively, there are ways of thinking yourself off the whirring hamster-wheel of fast heartbeat and fear, and convincing your mind to shift sideways into a calm and green land of happy thoughts.

Once I had a diagnosis of menopause and a bucket of HRT, my insomnia and anxiety lessened. Physically I felt better, but mentally I was still convinced that I was losing my face, my body, my personality and my brain, as well as my place in society as a functioning and useful participant. None of us are immune to the negativity associated with ageing generally and the menopause in particular.

A bloody quick global tour

Global experiences of menopause offer an interesting insight into how culture directly affects us. 'The social context in which a woman lives is important to her understanding and experience of the menopausal transition,' says Dr Sandra Thompson, Professor in Rural Health at the University of Western Australia.

Most studies, it's pretty widely acknowledged, investigate the experience of the white middle classes, which means our understanding is less than comprehensive to say the least. But there are some investigations which reveal staggeringly different attitudes. So, a 2007 study conducted in Guayaquil, Ecuador, found that 93.7 per cent of middle-aged women perceived menopause as a normal event, and that it gave maturity and confidence.[2] In taped interviews in Jordan, 2008, the menopause was seen as a positive transition, and a route to wise old age.[3]

Then there's the Hadza tribe of Tanzania, who are the ultimate example of positive old age. They are so frequently written about in anthropological studies that I'm surprised they are able to go about their normal lives without being interrupted every five minutes. They very much epitomise the Grandmother Hypothesis (see page 31), in that the older, post-menopausal women are useful within the tribe and contribute as much as the younger generation, foraging and giving away more food than they consume, as well as helping out with childcare. They are a vital and respected part of the tribe.[4]

> Respected for my wisdom?
> Not if you read Twitter after
> I've published a column!

My tribe, such as it is, consists of two teenagers, a hard-working husband, assorted relatives and excellent friends. To each I give different parts of myself (including food, especially to the teenagers, though I hardly forage), but I can't say I'm regarded as a wise woman by any of them. Useful? Yes, particularly when people want picking up from parties at three a.m. or need money for Uber fares. Respected for my wisdom? Not if you read Twitter after I've published a column!

What's most interesting is the fact that your culture's attitude towards menopause affects not just your feelings, but also your experience. Obviously, the whole period (or lack of them – that's almost a menopause joke) is also affected by genetics, lifestyle and – I strongly suspect – luck of the draw.

This has been flagged up for years. As far back as 1975, an

anthropologist called Marcha Flint noted that different cultures had different responses. She surveyed 483 women from the Indian states of Rajasthan and Himachal Pradesh, and noticed that most women suffered no symptoms of menopause. At the same time, she realized, once periods stopped, their quality of life improved. Before the menopause, women were expected to wear veils. Post-menopause, they were allowed to leave the women's quarters and publicly mix and joke with men. Might there, it was wondered, be a link?[5]

Later on, a massive 2015 study asked more than eight thousand men and women how menopause had affected their sex lives. Here, complaints were pretty much the same from Sweden to the States. But the level of difficulty in dealing with them differed, depending on how those countries viewed the menopause.

'In societies where age is more revered and the older woman is the wiser and better woman, menopausal symptoms are significantly less bothersome,' lead study author Dr Mary Jane Minkin, Professor in Obstetrics, Gynaecology and Reproductive Health at Yale Medical School, said at the time. 'Where older is not better, many women equate menopause with old age, and symptoms can be much more devastating.' She pointed me to a 2019 article she wrote on the subject. 'For many women, this change is liberating, freeing them from anxieties about childbearing, and from pain or discomfort related to their reproductive organs. Some women may view menopause negatively, associating it with ageing, which in most Western cultures has significant negative connotations.'[6]

Even vocabulary affects our perception. Dr Sandra Thompson was also the senior researcher on a 2012 study explaining that the language used around menopause can demonstrate how a society perceives a topic. 'Menopause in the Western world is largely medicalized, with much of the language being dominated by negative imagery such as "reproductive failure or ovarian failure",' the authors wrote. Clearly, the wording isn't designed to deliberately make you feel bad, but it's not exactly vibrating with positivity. 'In the Arab world,' it continues, 'the word corresponding to the menopausal and mid-life period means "desperate age".'[7]

So, if menopause is ignored or seen as a bad thing, it's going to make you feel worse about it. Unless you're given positive imagery and a sense of future advantages, it's no wonder that so many of us approach it with the dread steps of the condemned! How much better would our menopausal experience be if it was widely regarded as a new dawn on the horizon? People would be seeking us out for wise counsel and revering our longevity, wisdom and valuable contribution to their lives, instead of sniggering and going back to their mobile phones because you're just so, like, old.

To be honest, taking control of our thoughts and finding ways to lighten anxiety aren't just skills for menopause, they are skills for life. Our response to danger is what has kept the human race alive, but now that the sabre-toothed tigers are all gone, much of our sense of peril is self-created. Our negative thoughts can become – metaphorically speaking – the sabre-toothed tigers of the twenty-first century. If any of this makes you think, 'Aha! It *is* all in your mind, love,' then this is the wrong book for you. Take a time machine to the 1950s and live among *your* tribe.

Mind over matter isn't a new concept, but it's one worth investigating and, I'd suggest, rewording. Mind *with* matter is the ultimate collaboration, and one I consider well worth aspiring to achieve.

Start with CBT

HRT is not the only way of treating menopausal symptoms, and nor is it a wonder drug that alleviates every condition. To support it, and for those who don't wish to or can't take it, there are other therapies that can definitely help to negate the more debilitating impacts of hormone disharmony.

As I've said, thinking or breathing your way through the unavoidable ebbing of hormones was something I really didn't want to believe was possible. To say I was extremely sceptical before I made my 2018 menopause programme is an understatement. But then, as part of my research, I met five women who weren't able to take HRT and who all suffered from debilitating hot flushes, which had devastating consequences on their quality of life. I watched them going through a four-week programme of Cognitive Behavioural Therapy, or CBT, a talking therapy, at the end of which they had seen a sixty-four per cent reduction in hot flushes, and a ninety-five per cent decrease in the night sweats which affect mood and sleep. I sped from sceptic to full fangirl. The transformation in this group of hitherto suffering women was extraordinary; they radiated contentment and confidence.

> I sped from sceptic to full fangirl. The transformation in this group of hitherto suffering women was extraordinary; they radiated contentment and confidence.

This was all thanks to the work done by Myra Hunter, Emeritus Professor of Clinical Health Psychology at King's College London, and the co-author, along with Melanie Smith, of *Living Well Through the Menopause.*[8] She has devoted her career to exploring the possible links between what we think and how we feel physically, and is frustrated by the fact that, in our culture, everything is attributed to menopause at this time of life. 'It means that much of the information available – and especially online – are the extremes, so women unwittingly expect to have all the symptoms, enter this phase with dread and are therefore more likely to have a negative experience.'

'Remember that all pain or physical discomfort is to some extent affected by psychosocial factors.' By this, she means that, for example, should you experience chest pain, you'll instantly assume you're having a heart attack because that's what we've been led to believe. I can empathize with this; so much as a twinge in my ribcage, and

I'm sitting up in bed wondering whether to poke my husband awake so he can call 999, or leave him snoring peacefully and suffer quietly, alone, grumpy and, I suppose, possibly dying, although so far it's not happened.

'Eighty per cent of people who seek medical advice with chest pain don't have heart problems,' says Myra. 'Your reaction to chest pain will also be a stress reaction. This applies to the menopause, where symptoms can become a negative cycle. Just bear in mind that these are also affected by the ageist and the sexist views to which we're exposed.'

CBT is helpful for managing hot flushes and quality of life, and mindfulness and yoga are useful for general well-being, she tells me.

CBT is effectively a non-medical approach that helps people to develop practical ways of managing problems and offers coping solutions. It's so well proven that it is prescribed on the NHS – even making an appearance in that hallowed NICE guidance for menopause. You can ask your GP about it or self-refer.

What I love (now) about this approach is that it's fairly simple. So, if you are anxious and stressed, you are encouraged to write down your thoughts, feelings and reactions, and then consider whether they are overly negative. Look at your lifestyle; try to eat and drink sensibly, don't overwork, and don't avoid people.

Myra says that, if you're suffering a hot flush and worry about what people are thinking or noticing, it may make you feel self-conscious, impact on confidence, and also intensifies the feeling of the flush. 'If you are hot and sweating in a meeting, you may think everyone has noticed, and believes you're over the hill.' So true – those five women told me that they lived in a state of embarrassment. The flushes felt like an admission that they were getting old.

They had to put in some effort. There were interactive sessions and they were asked to put their thoughts and goals in a diary. They were reminded that even relatively small things can make a difference: improvements in well-being, such as reading a book before bed. I know this sounds patronizing; we've all read the women's magazines with listicles of 'how to have me-time', and rolled our eyes at the seemingly lazy repetitions of 'leave your phone downstairs' and 'have a warm bath'. But these tiny details are all worth considering and have honestly been an enormous help to me over the last few years.

'The women were also taught paced breathing, an exercise which involves slow, deep breathing from the stomach. The idea is that it may ease anxiety enough to alleviate the hot flush, or even stop it from being fully triggered,' says Myra. While I never suffered frequent hot flushes, paced breathing has been indispensable for me in helping to fall asleep again when I wake up full of anxiety four or five times a night, fretting about imperative details, like whether I wormed the dogs.

If you don't panic, or get angry and frustrated (easy to say, I know; my temper goes from zero to ten in a heartbeat, since menopause), and simply surf the rising heat in your body, then the flushes won't impact so much on your life.

The results were quite extraordinary, and because of the inter-active nature of CBT, it has the added advantage of being something you have personally achieved, lending a much-needed sense of control over what's happening to your body. It is true empowerment.

You will be pleased to hear that CBT is becoming more prevalent, and Myra is trying to make it easy to access, and even available to use online.

Yoga

Yoga is my other weapon against post-menopause insomnia, stress and generally seizing up. A handful of times in the last five years, I've gone to a retreat in Devon called Yeotown. Here, I walk, detox (sensibly – no caffeine, no alcohol, no sugar), and do yoga twice a day. Obviously, this is very much how I'd like to live out my life, but so far I seem to have become very easily distracted from that utopian model the moment I'm not under supervision!

It's hard not to gasp when you see what a lifetime's devotion to yoga practice allows the co-owner Mercedes Sieff to do with her forty-something body. Following her in a yoga class is like having Cuban ballet dancer Carlos Acosta teach you Zumba. The communal loo by the Yeotown kitchen is full of pictures of Mercedes doing handstands on paddle boards, and cartwheels on glorious north Devon sands. If you've got it, you must absolutely flaunt it. For those of us, like me, who don't, it sets the bar quite high. Our loo is full of pictures of me attempting similar moves at parties through the decades.

Watching Mercedes lead the class invariably makes me feel like a stiff and toxin-riddled hag. Nevertheless, after my five days on the programme (like rehab!), I always return refreshed, revitalized and determined to carry on with the good work, until someone plonks a steak and a glass of red wine in front of me and I embrace retoxing with gusto. When I'm low on energy, feeling peaky or over stressed, Yeotown helps me to reset. It's a glimpse of how much better we'd all feel without a full-time job, stress, kids, partner, commute and a love of refined carbs to boost energy levels rather than those 'power ball' fibre-filled alternatives.

Obviously, a few days at a luxury reboot camp like that is an enormous and expensive treat. When there's a chef concocting amazing gourmet vegan food, it's not hard to forswear normal temptations. On a day-to-day basis, eating like a Michelin-starred Rastafarian and summoning up relaxation techniques when confronted by life's hurdles is an impossible challenge. I still try to do yoga a couple of times a week, but ironically the days when I most need it are those during which I can't even find the time to make the bed before scooting out of the house. However, there's firm evidence and countless positive clinical studies highlighting the benefits of regular yoga for mid-life health, and it absolutely doesn't have to take place in five-star surroundings.

The physical postures and breathing exercises improve muscle strength, flexibility, blood circulation and hormone function, and the relaxation is beneficial for the brain. Once I started reading about the subject, I discovered that there are specific menopause benefits: yoga helps you to manage stress, anxiety and insomnia – all boxes I've regularly ticked on the symptom chart.

Yoga fans seem relaxed about the fact that you can call a class anything you like; there is anti-gravity yoga, where you hang upside down, laughter yoga (self-explanatory), and even dog yoga, where you writhe around your bemused hound. In that line-up, menopause yoga sounds positively pedestrian.

I am pleased to note that the teachers trained for yoga expert Petra Coveney's menopause yoga classes are mainly in their forties and fifties, and with experience of menopause.[9] 'I wanted women who were experienced teachers to feel that they had life experience and wisdom to share. I also have menopause yoga teachers in their twenties and thirties who have Premature Ovarian Insufficiency'.

> There is anti-gravity yoga, where you hang upside down, laughter yoga (self-explanatory), and even dog yoga, where you writhe around your bemused hound. In that line-up, menopause yoga sounds positively pedestrian.

'We talk about everything from hormones to sore vaginas, so it helps to have teachers with personal knowledge,' she says. 'I teach all round the world, including parts of Asia, Europe, Canada, the USA, and the Middle East, where we can't call my practice menopause yoga because of the cultural taboo. In all of these countries, women tell me that they feel alone, afraid and the hormone imbalance makes them feel as if they're going insane. Being able to talk to other women and practice yoga together (in person or online) makes a huge difference to their mental health and physical well-being.'

Her menopause yoga really took off in 2018, following the Everyday Sexism and #MeToo movements, when, as she says, women felt they didn't have to suffer in silence anymore. Classes are divided into three sequences, for perimenopause, menopause and post-menopause, as well as specialized movements for those with osteopenia (see page 108) and sleep problems.

Sign me up now! Though I do wonder if other post-menopausals like me ever pretend to be peri just for amusement. There is also research showing that, when women are stressed, we release oxytocin and seek the company of women for comfort. I can absolutely concur with that, whether I'm doing a downward dog at the same time or not.[10]

Mindfulness and meditation

I'm not a natural candidate for meditation, although I would probably benefit hugely from mastering something that puts boundaries around my brain's restless meanderings and my inability to sit still. Over the years, I've tried many different ways to make myself mentally stronger. I know that meditation and mindfulness are potent therapies, but I'm also aware that I need more discipline!

I may not be a natural meditator, but on the few occasions I've tried, I've felt calmer for the effort, even though I wouldn't call it Zen peacefulness. My mind is far too good at wandering off to deadlines and life logistics, or what Netflix option I'll go for that night, but, in the words of the famous (mindful?) advertisement from Tesco, 'Every little helps'.

A review of the available evidence regarding mindfulness (among other therapies) was published online in 2018. The positive thoughts of a study in *BJOG: International Journal of Obstetrics and Gynaecology*, published by our very own Royal College of Obstetrics and Gynaecology (RCOG), sound credible to me, though I object to their referencing symptoms as 'bother', as in 'Bother caused by hot flushes'. It feels very 1950s, though is frequently used in menopause studies. Personal irritation aside, they conclude that psychological interventions are a positive solution for menopausal women, and especially those who don't wish to or can't use HRT.[11]

But what *is* mindfulness? I've always vaguely thought of it as being an appreciation of birdsong. I asked Vidyamala Burch, expert and author of *Mindfulness for Women*,[12] to clarify.

'Mindfulness, on a personal level, has changed my life beyond all recognition, helping me accept and live with disability due to partial paraplegia. I know how powerful it can be, which is why I wrote my book and founded my Breathworks programme,' she says.

'At its most simple, mindfulness is awareness of what's happening in any moment, whether mentally, physically or emotionally,' she says. 'Once we know what we are experiencing in an immediate and direct way, we can then choose how to respond and live with more clarity and confidence. When we are not aware, it's as if we have a kind of fog surrounding us, a self-generated cloud of thoughts and feelings, worries and anxieties, that sweep us away and so often undermine and even torment us. Mindfulness helps dissolve this fog, so we can "come home" to our direct experience in any moment – what we see, smell, taste, hear and touch. We feel more vividly alive as we experience what is actually happening, rather than being lost in all our interpretations, fears and so on.'

This makes infinite sense, and tallies with what I understand as the simplest explanation of mindfulness: that it's appreciation of the moment. So, for example, savour your first sip of coffee in the morning, focus on the birdsong as you walk to work, and – quite literally – wake up and smell the roses. Try to experience every moment for what it is, rather than what you project onto it with negative thinking. If you stop and listen to the natural world, you can find your place in it so much improved. See and feel the beauty in the moment. And before you think I've floated off on a cloud of HRT-induced hysteria . . .

'I'm not saying practise this and have an amazing life,' Vidyamala says. 'There are always difficult things, but awareness builds resilience. The fear of what might happen falls away and you appreciate the present. Everything is pared back to what is happening now, and then the present moment blooms into richness.'

She says that she uses the image of direct experience as being like waves on an ocean. 'When awareness is shallow or light, you are like a dinghy being tossed on the waves. When your awareness of the moment is deep, you are a big yacht with a keel and mast. The waves are still there, but one's attitude is profoundly different.' To put it even more simply, it's mind training. 'We understand physical health and fitness: going to the gym and eating five pieces of fruit and vegetables a day. But there's no decent messaging about our mental health. What makes more sense than training your mind to work with you rather than against you? Training your mind with meditation can become as embedded in your daily routine as flossing your teeth.'

As an example of how it might work with the menopause, she says that, if you are panicking about having a hot flush and worrying about how you feel and how others are looking at you, mindfulness can bring clarity and calm. This is very much in tune with the CBT approach, which employs similar techniques.

Looking *at* your thoughts with perspective, rather than *from* your thoughts and being completely identified with them, can bring peace, for example, about the ageing process, which is so entwined with our fears about menopause. 'Be honest. You can recognize the current cultural assumption that you're becoming a wrinkly old lady, but you don't need to buy into it. Now I'm sixty, I've decided to adopt the wise old woman archetype and grow into it. I want more stillness and have less ambition. It's not bad, it's just different. You have a choice: you can fight getting old and hate it, or you can wonder how to embrace it and see it as an exciting and new rich phase of life. Anyway, who wants to be young again, with all the angst?'

> As a committed stress-bag, I know it seems unlikely that stepping off the treadmill for five minutes a day will have a beneficial impact. Isn't stopping just an invitation to let the balls drop? No, is the answer.

Clearly, Vidyamala's not had to fight against the ageism of television and radio, and actually, I'd give anything for twenty-four hours with my twenty-four-year-old face and body, just to understand with the benefit of hindsight how great it was then, but even so, she has a point. The bonus of mindfulness is that it's free, you can do a meditation in just one minute, although longer is preferable, and you can do it anywhere, although a peaceful location is more conducive to success. The more you practise, the better you become at being in the moment.

'Mindfulness can have rapid results, and with practice you can radiate calmness, which positively affects those around you,' Vidyamala tells me soothingly. Anyone who has met me will know that my natural default is slightly frenetic, as I attempt to do ten things at once. I am charmed by the idea that, with a bit of effort, I might radiate post-menopausal calmness.

Conclusion

As a committed stress-bag, I know it seems unlikely that stepping off the treadmill for five minutes a day will have a beneficial impact. Isn't stopping just an invitation to let the balls drop? No, is the answer. The most important thing I've learned on my own adventure is to remember that we have one body, one mind and one life. I can't help wondering whether menopause is also a reminder to women, who carry so much of the world on their shoulders, that we are not infallible. We need to stop trying to take care of everyone around us and try to take better care of ourselves. There is no harm at all in discovering how best you can press the pause button and breathe new life into your body. *Namaste!*

Three-Minute Meditation by Vidyamala Burch

Sit or lie comfortably and relax. You can be inside or outside.

Observe how your body feels: what physical sensations you're experiencing. Is there a cushion behind your back or underneath you? Simply notice the sensations for a few seconds.

Now listen to any sounds: loud, soft, high, low. How do you respond to them? Don't try to identify where they're coming from, but just listen. Allow the sounds to come towards you and allow them to flow around you. If it's silent, notice this.

How does your breath feel? What parts of your body are moving as you breathe? Try to be aware of these movements and the sensations of breathing from the inside, rather than as an onlooker.

Now move to your emotions. Are you generally happy, sad, calm or angry? Gently tune into your 'emotional weather' without harsh judgement. Can you have a bit of perspective on whatever you're feeling as you quietly sit with the experience of breathing?

Be aware of whatever thoughts are flowing through your mind. See if you can have perspective here too – let your thoughts be like clouds passing across the blue sky of awareness rather than statements of fact. Can you look *at* your thoughts rather than *from* them?

Finally, just rest in your body – being present in the moment, and noticing breathing, feeling, sounds and emotions as they happen. Let everything come and go with a sense of flow, moment by moment.

Breathe deep

Calm breathing tells the body that all is well, even if it's not. It soothes stress and anxiety and boosts the immune system. There is so much evidence about the positive benefits of breathing correctly that people have written entire books about it. This has been the cause of great hilarity in my house, with teenagers hooting with glee at the idea of grown-ups being 'so dumb' (not my words, obviously) that they can't even breathe properly.

Breathing Exercise by Vidyamala Burch
Do this whenever you feel it might be helpful.

Feel your feet on the floor and your bottom on the chair, if you're sitting.

Take a deep breath in, bringing your awareness into your abdomen and letting it swell out.

Let the out-breath flow all the way out, letting your abdomen subside back and giving the weight of your body up to gravity, so that it's supported by the floor.

Let the in-breath flow back in again in its own time.

If you can, let this embodied breath awareness be an anchor for the mind as you keep giving your weight up to the support of gravity with each out-breath. Allow your thoughts to come and go like clouds in the sky.

Meditation was my saviour

ARTIST ZOE GRACE, FIFTIES

Meditation saved my life. When I was forty-eight, my periods were all over the place, my breasts were massive and I was bloated. I felt unattractive and low for no reason. It was definitely my hormones. Then I did a three-day meditation course, and it was life changing; not like an amazing epiphany, but a gentle breeze. I spend twenty minutes every morning and afternoon meditating. You have your own mantra, and the deeper you go into your meditation, the more stress is released. My dad was sick at that time and my son was in his teens, but I handled it far better than I expected. Almost a decade later, I still meditate every day.

Forest therapy helped me de-stress

BESTSELLING AUTHOR OF *FOREST THERAPY: SEASONAL WAYS TO EMBRACE NATURE FOR A HAPPIER YOU* SARAH IVENS, FORTIES

On entering the perimenopausal phase of my life in my forties, getting outdoors and into fresh air and sunshine became the most crucial part of my well-being routine. Writing myself a green prescription and making a daily appointment with Mother Nature was sanity saving, allowing me to rest better, feel happier and blow away the cobwebs of exhaustion.

I am overwhelmed with medical research showing that this approach is scientifically proven and beneficial. Firstly, getting outside into natural light increases our levels of serotonin, the 'happiness hormone' that helps with many common menopausal complaints such as depression and headaches.

Being in the great outdoors also lowered my anxiety. Decreased anxiety and improved mood have been linked with walking in the woods; one study said that taking a walk outdoors ought to be prescribed by doctors as a supplement to existing treatments for depressive disorders.

The *Journal of Affective Disorders* released an analysis that declared how every green, natural environment (not just forests!) improved mood and self-esteem,[13] a crucial element for personal happiness, and that the presence of water, such as a lake, a river or the ocean, made the positive effects on happiness even more noticeable.

Many studies show exercising in forests – or even just sitting in one – reduces blood pressure and decreases the stress-related hormones cortisol and adrenaline, which helps us to calm down. Even looking at photos or drawings of trees has a similar effect – that's why the screensaver of my work computer is an image of California's Muir Woods. One study published in the *Biomedical and Environmental Sciences Journal* showed that even a view of nature out the window lowers stress.[14]

Just spending twenty minutes a day in a peaceful, beautiful spot – a local park, next to a river, going for a walk along a tree-lined street – really allowed me to improve my key symptoms of insomnia, anxiety and low moods.

CBT changed my life

NUTRITIONAL THERAPIST (TRAINEE) LYNN BRADBURY,
FIFTIES

Taking HRT is a personal decision, and no matter how bad my life, I didn't want to ever take it. But I knew I needed help. I watched Mariella's programme about the menopause and realized that CBT might be the solution. I'd had three or four hot flushes a day in my late forties and found that acupuncture worked. But then they went up to thirty or forty a day by my fiftieth birthday, and were perpetual. Cutting out sugar halved them, but even so, I was exhausted, my sleep was disturbed, my mind fuzzy and I felt as though I was burning out. I contacted the clinical psychologist Melanie Smith, who works with Myra Hunter, and they changed my perception and my quality of life.

I bought *Managing Hot Flushes and Night Sweats: A Cognitive Behavioural Self-help Guide to the Menopause* by Myra and Melanie and signed up for the online course, as well as three sessions over Skype with Melanie.

I did tasks week by week and my perception rapidly changed. Once you tell yourself, 'This hot flush will pass and you will be fine,' and wait out the sixty seconds or so, it just goes away again. It was a reality check. Apart from one guy who kept mentioning them, my co-workers were female and very sympathetic. I also realized that, even if you wake up a lot at night, you can still get through the next day.

I now have a list of triggers, such as certain hot drinks and flavoured crisps. I write a gratitude diary and do paced breathing and meditation. Now, I am retraining as a nutritionist. Incidentally, I get cold flushes as well. Nobody ever talks about those!

CHAPTER SIX

Meno-a-go-go: Diet and Exercise

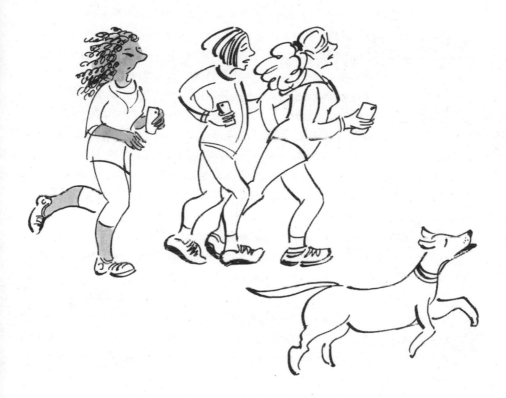

'At the age of fifty-two, I took up regular running.'

At the age of fifty-two, I took up regular running. Until then, I'd describe myself as having remained base-level fit. Then I reached that depressing moment in my thirties when taking exercise became necessary, rather than something I occasionally enjoyed. Walking – a love of trekking and pounding paths in the great outdoors – had always been my therapy. But in my thirties I supplemented this with going to the gym (the potential dating pool there was valuable in pre-internet-hook-up days!), and in my forties I realized that I needed to stretch out my compacting skeleton, and found yoga, which, along with daily dog-walking, seemed perfectly adequate.

Whatever stage of life you're at, making diet and exercise choices has an impact on how you feel physically and emotionally, as well as providing a template for future health. When it comes to menopause, the fitter and the more able you are to embrace healthy habits, the easier the transition is likely to be.

Mine may sound like a substantial commitment to exercise, but honestly it was low-level mitigation for a lifestyle that was otherwise stress-dominated, reliant on alcohol to relax, and punctuated by irregular meals based on convenient foodstuffs rather than nutritional value. Truthfully, my small-scale exercise regime had a lot to compete with on the retoxing front. But it worked for decades. I was slim, reasonably energetic, and seemingly silver bullet (the tequila-based cocktail) proof.

When I hit fifty, I hit a wall. A hangover would snake painfully around my head for twenty-four hours or more, and I started selecting nights I could let my hair down based on days when I wouldn't be working. It wasn't that I was drinking more, but the recovery period seemed to have doubled. The expectation of a late night also became a new consideration in my diary. I've never been a great sleeper, but now I was tossing and turning all night, with palpitations and anxiety, yet lucky to wake up any later than six a.m. That made the clock ticking anywhere close to midnight a Cinderella-style cut-off point for social activity.

Wondering why my body appeared to be failing, I did some research. The rather grim reading contained certain inevitabilities about women developing higher body fat, lower bone density, declining muscle and a fundamental physical inability to drink much alcohol, all of which are related to the two pillars of passing time: the menopause, and the natural process of ageing.

I realized that this was a time to be treated as a challenge, a mountain to be climbed. The only intelligent option was for me to face the fact that, like a boxer heading for a prize fight, aiming for peak health and fitness was going to be compulsory for my future. Sitting back and passively accepting decline would, I suspected, swiftly become a self-fulfilling prophecy. Appealing though it may seem, your fifties is not the time to slump onto a fireside chair and relax gently into old age.

To my horror, I discovered that lethargy can, quite genuinely, cause premature death. Prolonged sedentary behaviour in adulthood increases the risk of cardiovascular disease, type 2 diabetes and some cancers, and might be responsible for almost seventy thousand deaths a year. Adopting a sofa-based lifestyle could be costing the NHS more than seven hundred million pounds a year.[1]

Clearly, it was time to galvanise myself. With a bit of knowledge and willpower, we can most definitely nurture our bodies and minds for the future, which is more likely to be long and filled with excitement if you make a few lifestyle changes, regardless of how swiftly and easily you sail through the menopause itself.

I realized that what I'd taken for granted for decades in terms of health and fitness had now become an essential life goal. As much as we need to prepare ourselves mentally, rejecting the mythology that's kept us ignorant and afraid, and banishing all that bad messaging that's built up over the centuries, we also need to counteract and balance what's happening physically in order to battle the detrimental impact of declining hormones.

I firmly suggest that we take this as a 'knowledge is power' situation. Let's rise above the doom, and be grateful for the evidence confirming that, if we acknowledge the years around menopause as being a time to amend our lifestyles, embrace exercise and eat more fibre but less sugar, and consume less booze, we can set ourselves on a path to a more energetic and healthier future.

Don't bury your head in the sand. Look at your lifestyle and learn your family history, know your blood pressure and your blood sugar and cholesterol levels. Do what you can to boost your chances of a post-menopausal half century in the best possible health for you. Toast yourself with a small vodka and soda, the least brutal of poisons in my opinion, and bear in mind that it's never too late to make changes, whether you're in your thirties, forties, or your nineties!

Gravity, having children and years in sedentary jobs will inevitably take their toll. Whether to get your gloves off is a personal choice. My rallying call is to understand what's happening, take control of those challenges and determine to surf the waves with as much skill, expertise and style as can be mustered.

Basically, it's a good time to pick up the mantle of Dylan Thomas and, 'Rage, rage against the dying of the light.'[2] Although, in this case, the 'light' is our natural youthful energy and metabolism, rather than the grim reaper herself.

> Gravity, having children and years in sedentary jobs will inevitably take their toll. Whether to get your gloves off is a personal choice.

The hangover equation:
it's time to talk about alcohol

$$\frac{\text{Dehydration x Age}}{\text{Stress}} = \text{Sleeplessness} + \text{2-day headache}$$

Speaking as someone who once spent four days holed up at the Hotel du Cap during the Cannes Film Festival with a selection of debauched movie moguls *and* George Clooney, with barely an afternoon nap as sustenance, then went straight to work on Monday morning – you may know that imbibing Bacchus's finest is an activity of which I have some experience.

Now, though, I know that those happy decades when any problem could be diminished by a vat of fermented grape juice are well and truly behind me. Most women approaching their fifth decade and beyond will vividly recall the downsides of the fun: the horror of waking in the early hours and praying you didn't slur your words. Sleepless nights, miserable moods and puffy skin are all the enemies of elegant ageing.

The worsening hangovers are linked to age and hormones, yes, but also connected with levels of hydration, stress and sleep quality. Looking forward to arid, alcohol-free decades is enough to make any woman reach for the Chardonnay, but the truth is, it's time to cut down on the quaffing.

Does that mean that we have to become teetotal? Not necessarily. There are ways around this. In her book *The Hot Topic*, journalist Christa D'Souza wrote about embracing lower-alcohol wine – anything under eleven-and-a-half per cent.[3] My co-author, Alice, read this with great interest, as she – a lifelong dry white wine drinker – has found herself increasingly drawn to light and fizzy rosé wine.

I like the 'no drinking at home' rule, which guarantees most of us at least half the week giving our livers time off. Advanced non-drinkers will be able to graduate to 'not drinking during the week', though this can create a detox/retox mentality and terrible Sunday-night demons. Science is pretty clear that binge drinking is just as bad as daily drinking.

> But one lovely glass of red wine or a long, cool skinny bitch cocktail (comprised of vodka, lime juice and soda water), and I see my family in a far more benign light. They become charmingly bohemian rather than slovenly and irritating pigs.

For all the many downsides, I refuse to give up drinking completely. I'll tell you why. When I get home from a week in London on a Friday night, the house is usually a complete tip. The children's school uniform, or whatever they've been wearing, is laid out on assorted floors, like so many murdered bodies, as is an accumulated heap of wet towels. The dishwasher is full and dirty and chances of supper are 50/50, as my husband and I share the cooking when we're both around. This is clearly a highly frustrating state of affairs. But one lovely glass of red wine or a long, cool skinny bitch cocktail (comprised of vodka, lime juice and soda water), and I see my family in a far more benign light. They become charmingly bohemian rather than slovenly and irritating pigs.

Nutritional therapist Rayne Roberts says: make your choice – wine or whine

Menopause is a time to love your liver. And I'm afraid that goes hand in hand with mindfulness about your alcohol consumption. While menopause means that oestrogen levels plummet, what people often forget about the perimenopause is that oestrogen can go up as well as down – reaching levels as much as thirty per cent higher than usual. At the same time, progesterone – which usually balances oestrogen – is going steadily down. When this happens, your body tries to recalibrate by getting rid of the excess oestrogen, which is processed through your poor stressed liver.

Think about all the other pressures your liver deals with daily in the battle to detox your body. These include caffeine, chemicals in the home – even hairspray and perfume – and pollution outside. Throwing in alcohol adds extra duress.

As the years go by, alcohol, which is, let's not forget, poisonous in high quantities, has an increasingly toxic effect on the body. Age slows everything down, and that includes the rate at which you metabolize alcohol. This is because, during and beyond menopausal years, your body contains less water to dilute alcohol, and more (sometimes far more) fat, which retains alcohol.

Additionally, women produce less alcohol dehydrogenase, the enzyme that breaks down alcohol. This also contributes to higher concentrations of alcohol in female blood.

There's no question that it may exacerbate menopausal symptoms such as hot flushes, night sweats and lack of sleep. If you are feeling anxious and depressed, again, alcohol is unlikely to lighten the mood. And we all know the general dangers of drinking to excess: too much alcohol is linked to heart disease, liver disease, stroke, dementia and cancers, including breast cancer, and these risks increase as we get older. Oh yes, and alcohol is really bad for your brain, both long and short term.

Obviously, there are government guidelines about alcohol, but it's impossible to prescribe safe limits on an individual basis. The reality is that moderation is key. On the one hand, we know that alcohol increases the risk of breast cancer, but, on the other, there are studies proving the huge physical and emotional benefits of a glass of something with good friends.

SUMMARY: Be mindful. Enjoy the odd glass, but, ideally, this is the time to really cut down.[4]

The diet equation

$$\frac{\text{Fat} + \text{Sugar} + \text{Refined carbs}}{\text{Lower metabolism}} = \text{Weight gain}$$

Like most women, my weight has always been irrevocably tied in with my mental state. But that stops being an option as metabolism slows down. None of us can rely on meeting a new partner or getting a new job and instantly dropping half a stone.

It is a cruel time of life, when the woman versus weight-gain battle steps up a notch for us all. I struggled with yo-yoing weight in my early twenties, linked almost entirely to my turbulent emotional life. Happy and in love, I'd become waif thin; depressed and alone, I could gain five kilos in a matter of weeks. The real benefit of youth is how swiftly the impact of bad living can be negated. By your fifties, the ability to bounce back from bad lifestyle choices is not something you can rely on. That half bottle of white wine a day goes straight to your stomach and sets up home there.

For decades, my diet has kept me in a fluctuating but tolerable personal weight range. But then, in my early fifties, I began to pile on the pounds, particularly round my tummy, while my thighs became a road map of dimpled potholes. Having not really worried about my body or my health since my thirties (during my twenties I worried about everything), now I started to wonder if this was the beginning of the road to oblivion, and, truth be told, it felt a little premature.

It's tricky, because I have absolutely no truck with the majority of diets out there. From keto and cabbage soup, to maple syrup and apple cider vinegar, anything that involves elaborate menus, significant effort or dodgy science isn't for me. They also subscribe to a societal assumption that thin is aspirational.

I've learned that sugar in any guise is not my friend, and that it takes determination and commitment to compensate for unpleasant and sudden physical surprises, such as the inability to drop four pounds in as many days. As with puberty, we're back on an emotional rollercoaster. But, to make matters worse, comfort eating, slumping in defeat and dodging the world, as teenagers are wont to do, are no longer options.

You do need to eat in order to stay alive, of course, so that's a bit of good news. Even if you're lying in bed all day, three quarters of your energy requirement is being used up just keeping your heart beating, your lungs working and your brain thinking. Sadly, this doesn't mean you can lie in bed, not eat much and call it healthy living. What woman hasn't dreamed about a week doing nothing? Funnily enough, this is not what any experts recommend.

All this said, it's been pointed out by women far better than me that we need to stop equating being slim with somehow being a better person, and we need to stop always obsessing about being a few pounds lighter. Healthy, strong, happy and (reasonably) fit is far more important than dress size.

Rayne Roberts says: stave away the surplus

Many women reach their maximum lifetime weight during the perimenopausal years, when the average weight gain is five to eight pounds.

The reasons behind this are complex. Firstly, metabolism slows down as we get older. From our thirties onwards, we lose between three to eight per cent of our muscle per decade. Muscle burns calories with more efficiency than fat, so the more muscle you have, the higher your resting metabolism.

Oestrogen production declines as you head towards and beyond menopause itself. It's been shown that low oestrogen affects fat distribution – including visceral fat, the internal fat around the organs. For those who haven't changed their diet, be aware, biology is clever, and because fat makes oestrogen, your body stores more to boost your dwindling reserves.

During perimenopause, it's thought that fluctuating levels of cortisol and oestrogen may contribute towards weight gain: stress hugely affects hormones, so reducing stress levels is important.[5]

Finally, poor sleep can affect the hunger hormone ghrelin, and incline you to eat more.[6]

However, we also know that diets just don't work in the long term.

Short-term calorie restriction does have benefits, but, long term, women don't stick to diets, and besides, most of us aren't taking enough exercise. Fifty per cent of women are dieting at any one time, but being told to eat less is deprivation and very negative.

Your energy needs are likely to be less at this time of life, but I don't think that the oft quoted 'eat two hundred fewer calories a day' is especially helpful. It's more useful to be aware that small, regular diet-and-lifestyle changes may help.

Bearing all of this in mind, it's worth trying to eat the right foods! That means eating less sugar and refined products, and consuming more fibre in the form of fruit, vegetables and wholegrain carbohydrates. In a large study from Australia, researchers found that menopausal women who ate diets high in veg and fruit (and the occasional glass of red wine) were twenty per cent less likely to have hot flushes and night sweats versus menopausal women who ate high-sugar, high-fat diets. Why? Evidence shows that the high fibre content, which encourages gut motility (pooing, to you and me), helps excrete excess oestrogen and prevents it from being recirculated.[7]

If you repeatedly have high levels of sugar in your blood, your body releases more insulin to help it enter the cells and act as energy. If you keep producing insulin at high levels, you can become 'insulin resistant', which is associated with type 2 diabetes. Your cells ignore the insulin signals and the sugar remains in your blood, causing inflammation and encouraging the sugar to be stored as fat.

Women in parts of Asia, such as Japan, have fewer menopausal symptoms, and there's thought to be a link between this and what they eat. From an early age, they eat a diet high in soy – such as edamame beans and tofu. These soy-based foods contain phyto-estrogens, or mildly active oestrogens, in plant form. However, this lack of symptoms might also be genetic. There is some evidence that the Japanese have evolved with the ability to metabolize soy differently.

Having said that, it's worth trying to add more soy to your diet. A 2020 study pointed out that moderate intake of soy products is good for heart health.[8] And they also contain protein, fibre, iron and zinc. Soy milk in the UK is often fortified with crucial B vitamins, vitamin D and calcium.

Afro-Caribbean communities are more likely to eat diets high in yams, which are a source of plant oestrogens, or phytoestrogens, and are said to reduce symptoms. Yams are widely available in the UK, but the evidence that they help is mainly anecdotal. One study conducted in 2005 showed that twenty-four post-menopausal women replacing two thirds of their staple diet with yams had increased oestrogen levels.[9]

Healthy fats such as avocado, olive oil, oily fish, nuts and seeds are essential for everything: energy, cell function and helping the body absorb vitamins. A Mediterranean diet is one we could all follow, as well as ditching high-salt, high-fat and high-sugar processed foods, and reducing red meat consumption.

More than anything, you need enough protein. Firstly, the liver needs protein to function, and secondly, it's vital for maintaining that muscle mass.

It's recommended that women aim for 45 grams of protein a day, but I'd question whether that's enough as we age. It's not hard to include protein with each meal. A small chicken breast may contain 30 grams of protein, and there are 13 grams in two large eggs. Chia seeds make awesome porridge made with soy milk, a teaspoon of cocoa and a handful of frozen berries, and quinoa has the same amino-acid content as steak – swap out your pasta! A protein-rich breakfast is the best way of staying full throughout the morning, so do go to work on an egg.[10]

Finally, the gut is currently considered key to good mental and physical health. Recently, there's been a big buzz about the importance of our microbiome – the complex and vital community of bacteria and other bugs that live in our gut and are vital for our health. Our microbiome helps us extract vitamins and minerals from our food, and it also makes essential hormones and boosts immunity. It's even thought to be important for our mental health. The best way to feed our microbiome? By eating a very varied diet, full of high-fibre fruits and as many different vegetables as you can. It also loves fermented food, dairy containing live bacteria, and antioxidants, which you'll find in brightly or richly coloured food, including berries, chocolate and even coffee and tea.[11]

SUMMARY: Don't eat excess sugar, but do eat as wide a variety as possible of fruit and vegetables, and eat plenty of protein and healthy fats.

The wisdom of supplements

I can't help feeling that menopausal women are a gift to the supplements industry, as we can be both vulnerable and desperate. I have seen some quite extraordinary concoctions advertised, especially on social media, and with very strange sounding ingredients. These often purport to hold the secret to weight loss and amazing energy. Funnily enough – and I say this with heavy sarcasm – if you ask to see their clinical studies, they rarely respond.

> 'Don't be lured in by the massive market for mad-sounding menopause supplements.'

'Don't be lured in by the massive market for mad-sounding menopause supplements,' agrees doctor and presenter Dr Chris Van Tulleken. 'There is no robust evidence behind most of them for their ability to improve your menopausal years. In my opinion, women are being preyed on at a vulnerable time of their lives.'

That said, I do swear by certain supplements, which I've carefully researched. I take daily vitamin D, B vitamins, a probiotic, omega-3 and a hair formulation that my friend Gina Bellman recommended. This contains such hair helpers as zinc and selenium, and which I am sure has thickened my thinning locks.

Above all, I love magnesium. I generally have, within arm's reach, either magnesium spray, magnesium lotion or magnesium bath flakes. Do be careful not to overdose; I found that too much exacerbated symptoms.

My collection may appear to constitute product overload. But fellow sufferers of the debilitating condition known as 'restless legs syndrome' – problems such as joint and muscle aches and pains are common in menopause – will know that there are few lengths to which we won't go to banish the symptoms of this little-understood condition.

My attacks start with a slight fizzing in my calves that swiftly becomes a brain-addling desperation to stretch my 'restless' leg. When I was younger, it only struck when I was overtired or in cramped conditions. Plane journeys and nights at the theatre were particular triggers. Now, there's no accounting for when the tell-tale signs will turn a relaxing night's sleep into a marathon of irritated wakefulness.

Rather than restful slumber, I'm leaping in and out of bed to try and stretch. Yet, the minute I snuggle beneath the duvet, the symptoms return, often with a side order of agonizing cramp to make things even worse. A friend recommended I buy magnesium tablets a few years ago and, within a few days of taking them, the worst of my symptoms had eased off. But still, there were nights when I was woken at two or three a.m., the tell-tale ache in my lower calves making sleep an impossibility.

That's when I added spray to my shopping list, and it's become something of a miracle cure for me. Magnesium can be absorbed via the skin, and a quick squirt on the affected area before I go to sleep means the worst of my symptoms are vanquished. On nights when there's time for a pre-bed relaxing bath, I pop in magnesium flakes as well.[12] There are other reasons and treatments for menopausal aches in joints and muscles, but I'll stick with my solution.

Rayne Roberts says:

66 Supplements specific to the menopause are a very personal decision. On the whole, you should be able to get all your dietary needs through what you eat. But, let's face it, if we are busy, this isn't always possible.

Always check that whatever you take won't affect any medication you may be on. Supplements can have contraindications, and there's no guarantee that they will work for you. Some women swear by supplements which are on the market for helping with menopause symptoms. The problem is that they don't always have firm clinical evidence to back up their claims.

Make Sure You're Getting Enough . . .

VITAMIN D: This is the one supplement I absolutely recommend for everyone, and I've never tested anyone in my clinic and found they have optimal levels. The so-called sunshine vitamin is made by the skin when exposed to the UVB rays in sunlight. However, this is only possible in spring and summer; you cannot make it in the winter, and you can't store enough to keep you going through the darker months. Vitamin D is vital for bone health (it plays a key role in calcium absorption), immunity, reducing the chance of type 2 diabetes and for heart health. Official government guidance recommends we take 10 micrograms, the equivalent of 400 IUs (international units), daily between September and March.[13]

The critical thing about vitamin D in the UK is that, the darker your skin, the lower your levels are likely to be. Higher melanin acts like natural sunscreen to block vitamin D production. For example, it's been suggested that as much as ninety-four per cent of the South Asian population might be deficient in the winter compared to a suggested general average of twenty per cent. If you have darker skin, it's worth investing in a daily, year-round supplement. Some studies suggest that vitamin D reduces menopause symptoms, but these are not conclusive.

B VITAMINS: Found in wholegrains, meat, dairy, nuts, seeds, legumes and some fruit and vegetables, there are eight B vitamins – including B_{12}, B_6, folate and thiamin – and they work best taken together. Unless you've been diagnosed with a B_{12} deficiency, which means you need to take the single vitamin, it's best to take a vitamin B complex. They're great for energy levels and in times of stress when the adrenal glands are under pressure.

OMEGA-3: Probably only worth taking in supplement form if you aren't eating a couple of portions of oily fish, such as salmon, mackerel or sardines, every week. It has antioxidant and anti-inflammatory properties and has been shown to help with depression and hot flushes.

VITAMIN C: Found in fruit and vegetables, this is important during the menopause if you have bleeding gums. It's also helpful for joint and skin health. Vitamin C is essential for the production of collagen. If you eat enough, there's little point in taking a supplement, as you'll just wee it out!

MAGNESIUM: One of the most overlooked minerals, it's beneficial for anxiety, stress, muscle relaxation and aching limbs, and fundamental to both energy production and sleep. Found in legumes, nuts, avocado and tofu, magnesium deficiency is very common. It's been suggested that seventy per cent of us have low levels.

Menopausal Supplements

RED CLOVER: A source of natural isoflavones, or phytoestrogens, red clover may boost oestrogen in the body, with benefits to the heart, bones and menopausal symptoms. There's little firm evidence as to efficacy, but some women swear by it.

BLACK COHOSH: This plant mimics oestrogen in the body. Some studies have shown a reduction in hot flushes, others show no benefits.

SAGE: There's a little evidence for this common herb reducing hot flushes and sweats; a 2016 Iranian study with ninety-three women said that it helped with both. You can add it to lemon and hot water to make a tea.

GINKGO BILOBA: Extract from this tree dilates blood vessels in the brain so that more nutrients can pass into the grey matter. It's said that it may help reduce the brain fog which is common in menopause, and also contains phytoestrogens.

AGNUS CASTUS: This comes under various names and is widely used. It's said to relieve menopausal symptoms such as anxiety and hot flushes. There's some positive clinical research.

EVENING PRIMROSE OIL: This is taken by many women for PMT, but data is pretty low quality when it comes to menopause. It might possibly benefit some for night sweats, and there is some promising emerging data.

ST JOHN'S WORT: There have been some promising results from studies of this herb to treat symptoms of menopause; it may help with hot flushes, but is generally used to treat mild depression, anxiety and sleep problems. NICE points out that it may interfere with certain drugs, including SSRI antidepressants and medications for breast cancer. **"**

Don't be dense.
Thicken your bones and muscle up

To my surprise, I've become a middle-aged cliché when it comes to exercise. I am dedicated to finding the time for two or three yogalates classes a week via Zoom, as well as a couple of three-mile runs. I am sure that this maintains my physical and mental health. If I stop moving, my mood drops and my body stiffens up like an old twig. It's reassuring to hear experts say that, no matter how sedentary a life you've led, and no matter at what age you start to move a little more, you will benefit from working out. Even increasing the amount you walk is good for you.

> If I stop moving, my mood drops and my body stiffens up like an old twig.

However, it's only in mid-life that I've discovered that exercise isn't to be dreaded or done under sufferance, and it's about far more than just getting your heart rate up. Exercise releases endorphins – the happy chemicals that push the mind into a short-term euphoric state. Not only does this alleviate low mood and help with anger, but it has a long-term impact on positive self-perception. In addition, it's a great way of counteracting loneliness. My running has become as much about spending time with friends (being sociable is definitely good for mental health) as it is about trying to firefight the flab and my unstable fat/muscle ratio. What started as an effort has become a pleasure.

Exercise is also vital for maintaining and strengthening our muscles and bones. I am increasingly aware that these two go – if you will – hand in hand. Muscles support your skeleton, keeping you upright. Lose muscle mass and you become more likely to fall. I keep suggesting that we do our running with ankle, wrist or even body weights, in the form of gilets with weights sewn in. As yet, this genius suggestion on my part has been ignored by my naive (and younger) fellow athletes.

Like many women, I am haunted by the spectre of osteoporosis, or weak bones, which is one of the biggest health concerns for post-menopausal women. At the age of fifty, I had a series of medical investigations, including what's known as a DXA scan to measure my bone density. That's when I discovered I was osteopenic, where bone density is lower than average for my age, meaning that I was at risk of developing osteoporosis.

Back in 2018, I visited Dr Karen Hind, Assistant Professor in the

Department of Sport and Exercise Sciences at Durham University. She conducted an experiment with thirty menopausal women, none of whom were on HRT, to demonstrate the positive impact of exercise on your bones. I was pleased to discover that running, which I already enjoyed, was deemed one of the best forms of exercise for bone density. And, with a combination of HRT and exercise, I was able to reverse my diagnosis.[14]

Follow my lead, and jog on . . .

Dr Karen Hind says:

66 More than two million women in England and Wales are thought to live with osteoporosis, and the National Osteoporosis Guideline Group (NOGG) estimates it causes 536,000 fractures every year in the UK. But the problem with osteoporosis is that the first symptom is likely to be a broken bone. It's well worth being aware of the condition and the measures you might take.

As oestrogen levels gradually reduce, all women will experience some weakening of bone strength during perimenopause. You should be aiming to build up your peak bone density between your teens and thirties with good diet and exercise, and especially by doing exercises which also build strong muscle; this acts directly on the bone to develop bone strength.

After around the age of forty, bone density goes down very slightly, by around half a per cent a year, but when you hit menopause it drops very suddenly; women can lose as much as twenty per cent in the five to seven years post-menopause. This is because of the sudden drop in oestrogen.

Perimenopause is a time to focus on preventing this loss. It is difficult to achieve improvement in bone strength at this time, but as long as you maintain bone density and don't see any loss, then you're onto a winner. Exercise and HRT can both help to stave off that steep drop, as well as ensuring you take the recommended intake of calcium and vitamin D, which helps push calcium into the bones. If you have an early menopause, it's vital that you take HRT to protect bone density.

Caucasian and Asian women, who have finer bones, are more likely to develop osteoporosis. If you are Asian or belong to a community that covers up for cultural reasons, then a risk of vitamin D deficiency adds to the likelihood of developing it.

If you enter perimenopause with a strong family history of osteoporosis, it's probably worth asking your GP for a referral for a DXA scan. This is like an X-ray, painless, quick and will give you an indication as to your bone health; you may need medication or just to focus on good lifestyle.

Excitingly, we're starting to realize that post-menopause, when things have settled down, it is actually possible to improve bone density. Only certain types of exercise can help, and, in 2017, it was shown by an Australian professor that specific high-intensity exercises could help post-menopausal women with osteoporosis who had low bone mass. It needs to be closely supervised by appropriately trained exercise specialists.

Quite genuinely, every little does help. Go to the gym, walk, dance, do cricket, football and aerobics, and try to target the potentially fragile sites: the spine, hips, forearms and upper body. Our research showed that the oft recommended 10,000 steps a day was associated with improved bone strength. No matter how sedentary a life you've led, or at what age you start to move a little more, you will benefit. **99**

I walk it off

DAPHNE DAMACHI, SEVENTIES

I was actually put on HRT in my early fifties, in the 1990s, even though I hadn't noticed any symptoms. My doctor, who was on Harley Street, did some blood tests and then put a little implant under my skin. Most of my friends were on it, although we didn't speak about it. In spite of not having thought I needed it, I noticed a massive difference. I had so much energy. Then, after a decade, my doctor retired, and the new doctor said that, because we didn't know the long-term effects, I needed to come off it.

Now I do a lot of exercise – I love walking, and can still walk around Hyde Park. It is important to exercise and keep supple, so one of my benchmarks is touching my toes without bending my knees. I try to eat healthily, with lots of salads and spinach, and I still have great skin, but I think that's genetic!

I've altered my diet in advance

BEAUTY COLUMNIST FOR *MARIE CLAIRE*
DR ATEH JEWEL, FORTIES

In 2019, I had a (benign) lump in my breast and the doctor wrote a referral letter describing me as pre-menopausal. It hit me that I was starting to enter that time of change, and I didn't want to be defined by it. At least I now know that I am entering my perimenopausal years in the best possible health. Three years previously, there was a very high chance that my lifestyle would have killed me by the age of fifty. I was a workaholic and using sugar as my fuel. Although an incredibly healthy child and young adult, by my late thirties I was more than ten stone overweight. I associated food with emotion, and had gradually piled on the weight in direct response to childhood family trauma and work stress. When I was diagnosed with type 2 diabetes in 2016, there was no question that it was through my lifestyle. I gave up sugar and took up ballet and yoga, managing to lose seven stone within a couple of years. I still have two or three stone to go, but I feel infinitely better. I am currently borderline diabetic and, once the final weight is gone, I will have reversed the condition. Even more importantly, I've understood that reaching for the sugar was a way of dealing with negativity about myself. Now, I meditate or reach for colouring books or my yoga mat rather than sugary food.

CBD Oil

Dr Elisabeth Philipps,
clinical neuroscientist and CBD expert

CBD oil has been one of the biggest trends of the last decade and, I believe, rightly so. There aren't yet specific clinical studies into CBD oil and menopause, but the way it works in the body means that it can impact many menopausal symptoms, such as sleep, mood, memory, joint pain and even bone density. What's known as the endocannabinoid system runs throughout our bodies and receptors can be positively influenced by CBD oil.

There is good clinical data around sleep, showing that CBD oil both stabilizes and improves sleep quality. There's also good evidence to do with pain reduction, such as period pain and aching or stiff joints, which can often occur around menopause.[15]

One of the most exciting potential uses is regarding bone density. New data shows that it influences the system that prevents the breakdown of bone, meaning that there's potential for short- and long-term use.

Ensure you buy the right product. The manufacturer needs to be able to prove that their oil contains the amount of CBD they claim, and less than 0.2 per cent THC (the psychoactive ingredient), so that it's just a food supplement and won't make you high! There's a membership organization called the Association for the Cannabinoid Industry, which is relatively new. Companies listed there will be trustworthy (there are of course other good ones out there).

When dosing yourself, start low and go slow. A mouth spray absorbs the best. Start with two to four milligrams daily; in my clinical experience, most people end up on between ten and thirty milligrams daily. More doesn't necessarily mean more influence. It's generally fast acting. Negative side effects are anecdotal reports of vivid dreams, and there's potential for interaction with certain medications, such as beta blockers or antidepressants.

CHAPTER SEVEN

M-Ployment:
The Third Shift

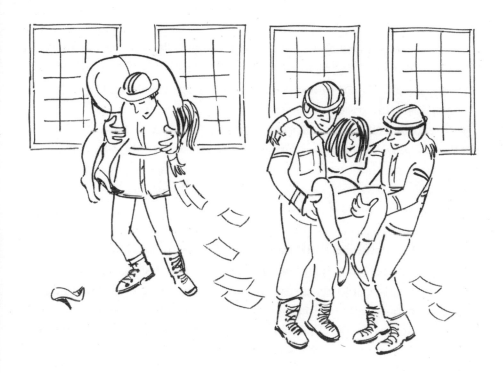

'There is a persistent picture in my head, which Helen Haddon, senior HR Partner at Derbyshire Fire and Rescue Service steadfastly refuses to indulge, of cohorts of handsome male firefighters nodding sympathetically during a menopause workshop, and then carrying all the women out, slung over their shoulders.'

If a cooling wind of change starts blowing through a woman's career during her late forties, it gets positively icy when she reaches her fifties. This might sound a rather pleasant meteorological phenomenon for those of us who are feeling too hot half the time. In reality, the metaphor is of little use. Age, up to a certain point, is described as relative, but as you approach mid-life it becomes depressingly defining.

There are around five million women aged fifty-plus in the workplace, according to the Office for National Statistics (ONS) statistics (and presumably the same sort of number aged forty to fifty, and – many – perimenopausal). Not that you'd know, given our lack of representation in so many areas of the advertising world, aside from pension plans, mobility equipment and funeral costs. With one in four likely to suffer severe menopausal symptoms, and many others struggling with less serious, but still significant ones, it's surely obvious that workplaces need to make provision for us and accommodate us better.[1]

A 2019 survey of 1,132 menopausal women by Newson Health Clinic revealed that seventy-six per cent of their workplaces weren't offering any sort of menopause support, in spite of over ninety per cent of respondents feeling that their symptoms were having a negative impact on work.[2] That's hundreds of thousands of us set adrift and on our own. The maths simply doesn't add up. We need a nationwide master plan to provide the same protection for women during menopause as we receive during pregnancy and periods of ill health.

The other day, I was talking to a female lawyer at a prestigious firm. When Katharine Hardie joined Pinsent Masons a couple of decades ago, they displayed a pioneering commitment to their expanding menopausal staff members by giving them an enshrined right to have the use of an electric fan. I'm not joking when I say this was pretty impressive stuff back in the early 2000s.

Katharine, not yet menopausal herself, and some of her colleagues became aware of many great team members who were suffering from confidence-eroding symptoms just at the point in their careers when they should have been benefitting from years of experience, and set up a pioneering menopause forum. 'The Fan Club' offered discussion and support, not just to stop the brain drain of excellent lawyers, but also to bring together all women in the firm and give them the opportunity to share their experiences.

Creating a space to have a conversation about menopause at Pinsent Masons has been instrumental in helping the well-being of a generation of women in the firm, giving a voice to many who felt unheard and retaining many experienced professional women who might otherwise have felt the need to leave their careers if they were not given the support and understanding they required.

Despite the increasing numbers of us in the workforce, in much of popular perception an ageing woman is still an increasingly redundant one, and it's an aspect of our working culture which is almost as stubbornly true today as it was in the 1950s. Back then, of course, what you lost at menopause was perceived as your only skill set – the ability to procreate. Now we're in the twenty-first century, it's insanity that our value as employees is in any way connected to our fertility.

There are many compelling reasons to have substantial numbers of female mid-lifers on the payroll. We're freed up from the demands of childrearing and the emotional rollercoaster of youthful relationships (who hasn't called in sick after yet another break-up?), but the effort and commitment remains one-sided.

If you're lucky, you get to hang on to your job, but turn up at an interview extolling the virtues of an enhanced skill set and a blast of incredulity is likely to blow you back out the door. I have witnessed first-hand how women in mid-life tend to be exceptionally hard and determined workers (at BBC Radio 4, where I worked for twenty years, they form the majority of the production teams, and do the bulk of the work). Undervaluing such key workers comes at a high cost to the British economy.

My working menopause

My own career history may be slightly unusual, in that I crawled back to my job within months of having both my babies. Much as I adored them, I struggled with the tedium of maternity leave after a full working life. Also, to be totally frank, as a freelancer with no prospect of maternity pay beyond the state's bare minimum, financial imperative also figured highly in my list of priorities.

Happily, maternity leave and your welcome back to work are enshrined in employment law, these days, and there are rules and systems in place to support you; whether these are enthusiastically embraced or provided reluctantly is of course another matter.

Back in the earlier part of this century, I did once get told, via my agent, that a BBC TV boss felt that my 'breastfeeding schedule' was not conducive to fulfilling my duties on *The Culture Show*, when I refused to commit to twelve-hour days. It's ironic that the reason the filming days were so elongated was because they were using graduates rather than professionals to direct the programme segments. Their lack of experience was illustrated by their need to reshoot over and over again. To my eternal shame, I did the 'honourable' thing and stepped down. Aside from that encounter with a tragically unreconstructed hierarchy, while at the *Observer* and Radio 4, where I worked for twenty years with an almost entirely female team, I always felt I was one of a gang trying to navigate the same terrain.

Further up the bureaucratic chain, I would be lying if I said the same were true. As I headed towards fifty, attitudes towards me started to change. Even with my skill set unquestionably improving with maturity, I stopped being considered for any of the coveted presenting positions that came up. Where once I was a name on the lists for *Desert Island Discs*, *Start the Week* or *Saturday Live*, I found that just hanging on to my regular book show was a challenge.

It was increasingly obvious that those in a position to promote me were wondering instead when I might gracefully accept retirement and remove myself as an obstacle to their pursuit of a younger listenership. Your fifties, it became clear, no matter how you dressed it up, were just not the right age for advancement, and especially if you were a woman.

When I wrote in exasperation to my then boss, his response was to ask in frustration why I wasn't simply grateful for my thirty-minute, three-weeks-in-every month, book show. The idea that I might have larger ambitions or want to work on a more full-time and challenging basis was clearly absurd. The expectation of gratitude for a job you have actually earned is yet another inequality between the sexes!

It is hard enough being an older working woman in an ageist society with a youth obsession. But if menopause robs you of your confidence and saps your energy for the battle, it's even harder to stop yourself being crushed by the tsunami of society's expectations. As increasing anxiety and sleeplessness in the couple of years from forty-nine to fifty-one took their toll, I found plenty of indignities and fears to flood my late-night subconscious and keep me from slumber.

At work, in a blur of sleep deprivation and assailed by mysterious symptoms of stress unrelated to the actual pressure I was under, there were moments when I was desperate to take a sick day. But what was my ailment? And, had I known it was menopause-related, would I have dared to highlight my condition? I've already discussed the less-than-supportive attitudes I encountered when I became a mother. Did I really want to throw myself on the mercy of those same patriarchal platitudes? Back then, I wasn't sure any woman had ever claimed a day off for menopause. For many women, the path of least resistance is the least confrontational choice, so they accept their fate, fade to grey and disappear from view.

I still suspect that a key reaction to a woman who has the temerity to be openly suffering from menopausal symptoms is sniggering and the nudging of elbows. That's why so many women find themselves paralyzed at the prospect of public humiliation, when hot flushes might turn them briefly into the crimson, sweating victims of hormonal imbalance. The thought of periods is still enough to make many flinch, but periods stopping because of age (yuck), along with being hot, sweaty, dry, agitated, exhausted and embarrassed . . . Well, it hardly bears thinking about.

It was almost a decade ago when my symptoms started, and happily there have been some improvements to the discourse and the conditions. Back then, there was no question of flagging up brain fog as a valid reason for taking a moment. However, to my surprise, our evolving attitudes to menopause at work might be one way in which the UK could be called 'world beating'.

This is not to say that the office is a Mecca of understanding, with open windows, quiet zones for a five-minute meditation, CBT instruction in controlling hot flushes, free fans on every corner and flexible hours for all. And there are still many examples of gross unfairness. But there is also brilliant campaigning, legislation, political engagement and a growing acceptance among all ages and sexes that menopause is something that simply happens, and that, as invaluable members of the workforce, women might need a bit of support.

> That's why so many women find themselves paralyzed at the prospect of public humiliation, when hot flushes might turn them briefly into the crimson, sweating victims of hormonal imbalance.

So, how *are* menopausal women treated in the workplace today, what are the changes that are taking place, and what further improvements do we still need to demand in a world that remains surprisingly resistant to creating a female-shaped professional space for working women? And, from a business point of view, is doing so – let's be blunt – going to make you more money?

The menopausal workforce: who are we?

First of all, we menopausal women are genuinely a force to be reckoned with. We're the fastest-growing section of the workforce. According to 2015 data from the Department of Work and Pensions, the biggest increases in employment rates over the last thirty years have been for women aged sixty to sixty-four (from eighteen to forty-one per cent) and for women aged fifty-five to fifty-nine (from forty-nine to sixty-nine per cent). The Faculty of Occupational Medicine's (FOM) guidance on menopause and the workplace highlights that nearly eight out of ten menopausal women are in work.[3]

So, we are, like it or not, vital cogs in every wheel of the economy. Also, we need to work to pay the bills, as pensionable age seems to be slipping further and further down the line.

You're unlikely to miss gender inequality as you head towards the top of the tree, and, as you ascend to elevated heights, smashing glass ceilings as you blue-sky your ass into the boardroom, you'll more often than not find yourself awash in testosterone.

A rather magnificent piece of research called 'Woman Count 2020' was conducted by gender-diversity consultancy, the Pipeline. They found that FTSE 350 companies that had at least thirty-three per cent female membership on their executive committees had a net profit margin of 15.2 per cent, while those with no women had a net profit of just 1.5 per cent. That means that firms with no women on their executive committees missed out on forty-seven billion pounds in a year. So, more women = more money. In the words of that over-quoted, but genius, hair advertisement: we're worth it.[4]

Sadly, not everybody sporting M&S menswear recognizes the value of employing a vagina rather than a penis (or ignoring the whole appendage situation and going on merit alone). That's all sexism in the workplace comes down to, unless the suit in question is also employing on the basis of what friends you have and which esteemed school you attended. Here, I know that men also feel the injustice of the assumption that wealth and social class equals brains, and that speaking without a regional accent equals ability to lead, which I think we all know is untrue.

I say all of this as someone famed and employed for my own voice. But I am very much penis free, and my husky tones were honed in a series of Irish state schools rather than any high-end educational establishment.

This brings me to the next swathe of statistics from the same report, which contradict all of the above, when it comes to sense and meaning, and make you wonder if there really is a wilful conspiracy among the patriarchy to keep us in our place. In the three hundred and fifty biggest British PLCs, fewer than two in ten chief financial officers are women, only four per cent of investment managers are women, and just five per cent of firms are led by a female CEO. In the FTSE 100, there are more CEOs named Peter than there are women in the top job.[5]

In 2016, and apologies for the reams of statistics, but they fit together like a thousand-piece jigsaw and are building up to a crescendo of a conclusion, it was said that one in four women had considered leaving work because they couldn't cope with their menopausal symptoms.[6] As my kids say, charmlessly, and without looking up from their phones, *you* do the math. There is clearly a need for support.

A lot of the research we read to provide you with this information was eye-wateringly dry in tone, unless you are passionate about HR, which, thankfully, many people are, otherwise we'd probably have no workplace rights at all. But it seems quite evident that, from an employer and employee perspective alike, the menopause needs to be acknowledged and respected in the workplace. Like food for hungry children, it shouldn't have to be argued. If you're a business, it makes financial sense to look after your employees, no matter what hormones govern their health.

> Just five per cent of firms are led by a female CEO. In the FTSE 100, there are more CEOs named Peter than there are women in the top job.

What are the problems?

An Ipsos Mori poll in October 2020 found that half of working women aged forty to sixty-five have experienced three or more menopausal symptoms while at work.[7] As we know, many of the trickiest symptoms are also the most subtle, such as anxiety and brain fog. If these occur in the office – forgetting things or worrying about completing deadlines – it's hard to know whether it's just life stress and general pressure or a pesky period of hormonal change. Or both.

I am writing this book aged fifty-eight. Having worked since the age of sixteen, I have been peri- or post-menopausal for around a quarter of my working life. Yet, despite some pretty desperate days, following nights of palpitations and insomnia, and the low mood that often comes with lack of sleep, I've never once had a day off to facilitate my menopause. That's not a boast, it's a lament for me and the millions of women out there who struggle through debilitating symptoms, while juggling their domestic and work responsibilities and trying to look as youthful as possible so nobody notices they're middle-aged.

Hot flushes make it easier to identify what's happening. But a surge of red-hot heat rippling through your body as soon as you are stressed means that having a meeting or making a presentation in a room full of colleagues is pretty daunting. The all-consuming fear is that you'll wind up highlighting the very thing you're trying to disguise.

Few of us are comfortable sharing with a male line manager that they might need someone else to do the presentation to the new clients, for fear of fuelling the idea that women aren't able to do a job as well as men. The debilitating symptoms might be taking their toll, but does it sound credible, let alone professional, to be excusing yourself from work because your hormones are in turmoil?

Before menopause educator Deborah Garlick held a seminar with a Midlands police force in 2018, her company received a message from a female officer. 'She asked us to stop talking about menopause. They felt that it made them look weak, when they'd fought hard for equality.' This is one of the biggest fears behind addressing it in the workplace. Women may make up forty-seven per cent of the UK workforce, but acknowledging the fact of the menopause might make us look less employable.

'There's huge concern about women being seen as a bit ditzy,' says Deborah. 'In fact, we're working harder, if anything. Nobody wants to be patronized. They just want to do their job well, and that might mean minor adjustments to hours or environment. Too many of us still have the mindset that menopause is towards the end of life and career. You don't want people to think, "Oh, she'll be retiring soon." In reality, women take on more, compensate for their perceived "failings" such as tiredness, work harder and end up miserable. That's what we're trying to counteract.'

A 2019 CIPD (the professional body for HR and people development) report reads as follows: 'By taking the menopause seriously and treating it as an occupational health and people management issue, organizations can help to mitigate the potential negative impact of symptoms on the individual and the organization.'[8] That's it. Symptoms are something that may affect work and quality of life. So they need acknowledging and tackling, if necessary. It's so simple.

Breadth of support

Here is where the UK can give itself a round of applause. We are in advance of the curve – to use management speak (I think) – when it comes to menopause support in the workplace. 'The UK is further ahead on this than most other countries,' agrees Jo Brewis, co-author of an excellent 2017 government report about menopause,[9] and also Professor of People and Organizations in the Faculty of Business and Law at the Open University. 'An extraordinary number of organizations in the private, public and voluntary sectors are being reached.' Yet we need a hundred per cent of employers to offer training and support, so that's bad news for the rest of the world, who aren't doing as well, and hardly cause for celebration in the UK, where the number of women who've told me they felt in any way supported in their workplace is . . . zero!

I genuinely assumed that traditionally male-dominated job sectors would be incredibly resistant to education about women's problems, but – and I suspect there's a certain amount of arse-covering going on – this isn't the case. And, to be completely fair, it sounds as though seminars and talks on the subject are being taken seriously.

'It's a drum beat which is gaining momentum,' says Deborah Garlick. Her company, Henpicked: Menopause in the Workplace, reached over one million employees between 2019 and 2020, training them on the subject of menopause, which is a reassuring statistic. She has just launched official menopause-friendly accreditation for companies. 'Being menopause friendly is beneficial to employers and employees.'

Menopause trainer Julie Dennis runs similar workshops. 'It's a myth that men aren't interested in the subject. I think they're scared of saying the wrong thing and that a menopause seminar is going to be a man-bashing session. Every woman had to bring a male colleague to one session I did, and you could pretty much see the fingernail marks on the wall. However, during the course of the training, they became more comfortable, informed and open to talking about it.'

Then there's firefighting, a hot enough job at the best of times. There is a persistent picture in my head, which Helen Haddon, senior HR Partner at Derbyshire Fire and Rescue Service, steadfastly refuses to indulge, of cohorts of handsome male firefighters nodding sympathetically during a menopause workshop, and then carrying all the women out, slung over their shoulders.

Joking aside, Derbyshire Fire and Rescue Service has done a

sterling job of sensibly implementing measures to support meno-pausal women. 'Female firefighters are working till an older age, with the added pressure of having to maintain a certain level of fitness and in a male-dominated environment,' she tells me. Here, again, women are worried about being seen as less able or needing special treatment, which is why they're reluctant to come forward.

There isn't always access to facilities, but in Derbyshire they asked women what would be helpful and put simple practices in place, such as information on their intranet, menopause workshops and workplace champions, to whom women could speak in confi-dence. 'We've found that the more people understand, and that includes men and younger women, the more supportive they are. It's just something else to acknowledge as part of the working environment,' says Helen, in an example of the sensible, myth-bypassing and non-hysterical approach, which needs embracing on a national level.

Politics and end of periods

Even in the austere, male-dominated corridors of Westminster Palace, there is, if not exactly a fresh wind of change, certainly a hefty draft of possibility. Menopause is being, if not embraced, at least discussed. Tory Member of Parliament Rachel Maclean, then (in October 2020) Parliamentary Under Secretary of State at the Department for Transport, and who was instrumental in the deci-sion to make menopause part of the school curriculum, tells us that flying the end-of-periods flag in Parliament was a decision she didn't take lightly.

'I had to think very hard about whether I wanted to be the MP who talked about the menopause,' she says. 'Then I thought, Well, if nobody else is, who will? It's not a bandwagon everyone wanted to leap on. More of an "Oh God, really?" sort of subject. There was a reluctance to throw myself into it and make speeches. But then I discovered a statistic. Menopause had been mentioned some ridicu-lously small number of times ever in the history of Hansard. I looked at that and just thought, This is absolutely crackers. I can't live with myself if I don't do something about it.'

Hansard – incidentally – is the official report of the debates of both houses of the British Parliament, and which has been recording since 1803. We looked up 'menopause' in May 2021, and there had been 197 references (*ever*!) and four debate titles recorded about the subject. To put this in context, there had been 8,904 references to and 214 debates recorded about hunting, which is hardly relevant to five, never mind fifty per cent of the population.

Thankfully, Rachel did campaign for menopause education in schools (among other things) and she says that the then Education Secretary, Damien Hinds, embraced the idea, which was implemented in 2020.[10]

At the same time, Rachel was suffering from crippling menopause-related migraines, which were unresolved when I spoke to her. She says that she did what most women do: stay quiet and carry on, rather than speak up about her own suffering.

> Even in the austere, male-dominated corridors of Westminster Palace, there is, if not exactly a fresh wind of change, certainly a hefty draft of possibility. Menopause is being, if not embraced, at least discussed.

'My migraines coincided with my being elected as an MP. They hit me like a bolt from the blue and were totally new. Do I lie down? I can't. I'm a government minister. I'd love to be able to take a few hours off, but I have to go in front of the Transport Select Committee. I have medication, and I think, in all the time I've been a minister,

I've pulled out of things twice. The rest of the time, I just dose myself up, carry on and pray for the day to end. Menopause isn't cancer or heart disease, and in this job there's no way you ever want to admit that there's anything wrong with you, because of the environment, as I'm sure you can imagine. It's tantamount to saying that you're over the hill and you're weak.'

She is emphatic that menopause isn't a party issue, and in fact much of her work was with Carolyn Harris, Welsh Labour MP for Swansea East and Deputy Leader of Welsh Labour (in March 2021), who has overseen House of Commons menopause workshops held over Zoom, which were, she promises, attended by both men and women. Here, for once, it is me being the sexist one.

The thought of, say, Jacob Rees-Mogg listening intently to descriptions of declining oestrogen and nodding sagely, as though it was a particularly interesting Brexit point, makes me snigger. But Carolyn insists that the men from all political parties were respectful and interested. So shame on me.

Originally, they were going to have a fitness expert and dietician speaking as well, but at the time the nation was in lockdown with COVID-19, so plans were thwarted. Nonetheless, Carolyn says that they talked about the male menopause – a subject about which I have mixed feelings – and how you inevitably gain weight in middle age however much you exercise, with which I can absolutely sympathize. 'We've all got fitness bands and we have an exercise class every week via Zoom.'

I am glad that those who lead the nation are going to set an example, work out and look after their health. The sight of MPs taking time out from PMQs (Prime Minister's Questions) and trotting around Parliament Square in their Adidas tracksuits at lunchtime, checking their Fitbits, will definitely lend some much-needed comedy to our lives, much like Boris Johnson's born-again jogging commitment post-COVID. It could be the new Changing of the Guard.

In 2019, there was a push by MPs for a menopause policy. Carolyn Harris said at the time, 'You wouldn't dream of having a workplace where people weren't entitled to certain things because they were pregnant, and it's exactly the same for women with the menopause.

I firmly believe there should be legislation to make sure every work-place has a menopause policy, just like they have a maternity policy.' This sums it up for me. It's a basic right.

Harris's own experience was quite a difficult one, with years of heavy bleeding, followed by a collapse, the discovery of fibroids and then what appeared to be depression.

Her concern is that a lot of women appear to try to self-medicate through menopause. 'I think it can be a trigger for addiction; I've met quite a few women who've turned to gambling, alcohol and drugs. Three of them have ended up in jail.' She is hoping to get someone to research this. Having read research showing that times of high oestrogen makes us more vulnerable to addictive behaviour such as binge drinking, I can well understand this.[11]

Mental health help

In many ways, the emphasis on mental health awareness has helped the menopausal cause. 'Managers have been getting to grips with supporting workers with mental health issues for years,' points out employment lawyer Jog Hundle. 'They know that they need to step outside their comfort zone and what they personally understand, without making judgements.'

There is fear around the negative publicity of menopause shaming in the workplace. The age of social media and constantly being in touch can be blamed for many things, but it's a positive influence when it comes to colleagues knowing about poor workplace practices. 'Employers are judged if they don't look after their staff, and that's even more important than remuneration in terms of retention. It looks bad if they don't recognize that women need support,' says Jog.

'The number of women who hold senior positions around the age of fifty is getting higher and higher, and employers don't want to lose these skills,' adds Jog. (Incidentally, it costs thousands to replace an employee; I don't think this is entirely selfless.)

So sue me

If you're worried about maintaining your position at work, it's not all bad news. There are laws in place to protect menopausal women, even if they aren't specifically for that purpose (yet). Firstly, there's the 2010 Equality Act. There are nine elements to this, and Deborah Garlick tells me that menopause comes under three: age, sex and disability discrimination. Then, there's the Health and Safety at Work Act, which makes it a requirement to look after the well-being of employees.[12]

There have been a few tribunals where companies have been successfully sued, but it's impossible to quantify, as most will sensibly settle out of court. So, technically, if you're feeling in need of backup, there's a structure in place to give support, and education and awareness is increasing. You have legal rights.

Of course, as ever, it's those at the bottom of the money tree who are the most likely to suffer – working cash-in-hand or on zero-hours contracts, and therefore with fewer rights. Miss a day's work, and that might be the end of your time as a caregiver or support worker.

'I'm a white middle-class woman in my fifties, in a senior position,' says Jo Brewis. 'I've a lot of autonomy and have worked some of the time from home for years. Where you are in charge of your own diary, you can adapt.'

But the gig economy is, she points out, heavily populated by women, as a way of gaining the flexibility to support domestic lives where they are frequently still the predominant caregivers, and that means there's little protection for rights. 'Such women are dispensable. In fact, although legal protection exists and successful employment tribunals have been brought to safeguard these rights, employers don't tend to offer the same rights to all of their workers.'

The third shift

Isn't there – and you may have been thinking this for a while now – a bit of an argument emerging for simply not employing menopausal women? This attitude is a concern that has been voiced time and again by the experts to whom we've spoken, and it's certainly at the back of many women's minds when they worry about whether to communicate any health issues they are experiencing to their work-mates or bosses.

Jo Brewis says, 'Employers are well aware that if you treat a pregnant woman or new mother differently, then you had better have a very good excuse. It is correct to say that raising this issue does risk char-acterizing women. But the message is that menopause isn't that big a deal for most women. There's certainly no clear picture suggesting that menopausal women are falling off a cliff in an attempt to keep up.'

What worries her is that menopause is another shift – the third shift – after work and the jobs at home. It can be another burden. 'If women are suffering, then why on earth ought they feel they need to conceal it?'

Equally, there ought to be more research done into men around this age. Whether or not you accept that there is a male menopause (and I personally think that the evidence is scant, to say the least), there are still health issues; and this is a time of life when men ques-tion their choices, in the famed mid-life crisis – something which most women simply don't have the time or the income to indulge, in spite of having far more reason to do so.

As Carolyn Harris says, 'I still don't think current legislation covers menopause adequately. It's not us who need to adapt, but the workplace.'

I couldn't agree more. It's at the heart of why I embarked on this book. Menopause needs to be acknowledged, accepted and mitigated for, where necessary. Even more importantly, the value of mature, professional and committed women in the workforce, eager to throw themselves into new challenges, needs to be recognized, celebrated and embraced.

We are not a bunch of tragic harpies who can be shoved aside to allow for new blood (and dominated by the same old white men). We are a force to be reckoned with, for which there is compelling economic evidence, and, until society fully recognizes us, we need to be proud and strong and use our voices to demand change. A hot flush at the wrong time needs to be something we laugh off and learn to breathe through, not something we consider a shameful episode that keeps us awake worrying in the dark hours.

A first step we can all take to de-stigmatize menopause is for every working woman experiencing symptoms to say so out loud to colleagues, at least once a day, until the word 'menopause' itself loses its power to provoke judgement.

We may be improving, but that Ipsos Mori poll I mentioned at the beginning of the chapter (see page 171[13]) said that only around one in twenty women aged forty to sixty-five and at work is aware that their employer might be offering proactive policies or support. Seven per cent were offering a menopause support group and just six per cent access to specialist advice from an expert third party. Only six per cent of women said their employers offered their line manager or others a training course to increase menopause aware- ness. In conclusion, and if I were a teacher marking the UK, I would give a B- and the encouraging comment, 'Could do better.'

> In conclusion, and if I were a teacher marking the UK, I would give a B- and the encouraging comment, 'Could do better.'

Solutions

In 2016, the Faculty of Occupational Medicine summed it all up, and the solutions suggested are practical: ensure that employees and line managers are trained; encourage discussion, consider uniforms, flexible working hours and access to loos, drinking water and rest rooms; think about temperature control and generally offer advice and information.

The overwhelming evidence is that women want to feel that others understand what they're going through, even if employers don't *do* very much. 'This goes an enormous way towards feeling less scared and paranoid,' says Jo Brewis.

How to Approach Your Employer

DEBORAH GARLICK SAYS: We do recommend that women talk to their GP if they're struggling with symptoms.

Then the conversation with line managers is: 'This is what I'm experiencing (menopause), this is what I'm doing about it (looking at how I can manage my symptoms with my GP) and I'd appreciate your help at work with . . .'

When we're training line managers, we encourage them to ask if the woman has spoken to her GP. We know so many women don't get help and support, and line managers do need to know what someone is doing to manage their own health if they're asking for reasonable adjustments or changes.

Menopause in the men's room

EX-CHIEF CONSTABLE OF THE NOTTINGHAMSHIRE POLICE
FORCE SUSANNAH FISH, OBE QPM MBA, FIFTIES

Some women scamper through menopause and others have the most dreadful time. We implemented menopause policy in the force at the back end of 2016, which sounds recent, but, in menopause years, that's a very long time ago.

It helped that, earlier that year, we were the first police force in the country to bring in misogyny as a hate crime, and it changed the tone generally. In training sessions, men would say to their female colleagues, with genuine bemusement, 'But you're the first into a fight, you take no shit.' They would reply, 'Try being a woman. Ask your wife, your sister and your friends.'

One reason why I was able to make changes is that I was at the top of the organization; there is a command-and-control mentality in the police force, whereby, if you're told what to do by someone in charge, you do it. I had the leverage to make a situation happen.

The second was that I was a woman of a certain age, so I could empathize. The trigger was when a detective whom I've known most of my service came to see me for an exit interview. She wasn't at the maximum pension age, and usually police don't leave early. But her story was heartbreaking. She was having a difficult time with menopause symptoms, and when she spoke to her line manager she was simply told to 'get on with it', and dismissed. All she wanted was a bit of understanding and accommodation. Instead, she retired early. We lost a fantastic police officer with great skills and empathy.

I started to notice that menopausal women were all around me, in the way that you notice other pregnant women when you are pregnant yourself, and realized that there was a need for change. When I joined the force, back in the 1980s, women served for seven years on average and then left. Now, it's thirty-five years, and most of us are seeing through service in a similar way to men. The workforce is older, and women in their forties and fifties are at the peak of their careers, or heading towards it. In 2016, we weren't recruiting because of government cuts, so we needed to look at the economics. It costs thirty thousand pounds to recruit and train each individual officer, so there was a business case as well as a moral one.

Much against the better judgement of my head of comms ('Sue, we do murder and robbery'), we started to do some work around the message that every woman – whether black, white, gay or straight, and any class – would go through the menopause in some shape or form. A seminar we ran had some male attendees, and one of our chief officers spoke – actually, he completely outed his wife's experience, possibly not that appropriately. He clearly thought his response had been brilliant – I'm not so sure about her feelings.

We decided that information and support needed to be available to officers, and staff and working conditions needed to be reviewed. For example, one station was in a local-authority building where nothing was allowed on the desks, not even fans. It ended up with me having a bit of an up-and-down with the person in authority there, which I won. There was no good reason for the policy, in that context. We looked at uniforms, wondering whether they worked in practical terms – not just for foot patrol, handling dogs and guns, but also for hot flushes.

The police force loves a risk assessment, so we introduced one in terms of menopause. It meant that line managers needed to comply and think about it.

Some women, especially those higher up and accustomed to being in a male environment, were resistant to the changes, pointing out that it gave men another stick with which to beat women. But, actually, we have a leadership as well as a personal responsibility, and menopause affects us all. Senior officers often had wives experiencing it, and we pointed out to younger, more front-line officers that they could be better sons and daughters by recognizing menopause.

The workplace situation is improving and relatively positive, but there is still a long way to go.

Millennium: we were indifferent to the menopause

SARAH BARBER, FIFTIES

Twenty years ago, I was working in HR in the City. I honestly didn't think at the time that it was a misogynist environment. It was certainly male-dominated, and the majority of women worked in clerical jobs, with the senior positions being occupied by men. I wouldn't say that the few women with more senior titles were seen as ball-breakers exactly, but there was definitely a tendency for the men to tease us for being 'bossy' or 'not being able to take a joke' at times, which of course is sexist. It was a fast-moving environment and there were big changes afoot in moving from paper to electronic systems. Fewer staff were needed and those remaining needed different skill sets. As the majority of the clerical staff were older women, this affected them disproportionately. They appeared to lack the ability to learn the new methods, and often ended up making way for younger women. Now, I wonder whether we were being ageist – in assuming that women in their fifties wouldn't be as open to change.

The need for change

CHIEF EXECUTIVE OF CHANNEL 4 ALEX MAHON, FORTIES

I had not realized how impactful and dreadful the menopause was in women's lives until my eyes were opened to it by a couple of women I know in their fifties and sixties. And then I realized that utterly brilliant and experienced, and thus very valuable, women were leaving the workplace because of a health problem – albeit a temporary and fixable health problem, and one we will all experience. And that the onset of the health issue was coinciding with caring pressures, sometimes happening far earlier than expected, and often coinciding with a real and common life stage where one wonders if one is still attractive. This stage is hard for men too and is notoriously often tackled for them with a Porsche/golf trip/second wife. But it isn't even talked about for women because of embarrassment and shame, and a somewhat pathetic lack of ability to address issues to do with women's health in our conversations.

And then this seemed a pointless, unfair and discriminatory perspective, and one I noted was a real taboo in the workplace. An utter taboo. A pointless taboo. And I thought that that kind of discrimination isn't right.

I realized we could make a big deal about it and get big coverage (I didn't clock quite how big!) if I announced it all as a female CEO, and I realized that, in doing so, lots of people would make assumptions about my age, or ask me if I was in early menopause, if this was personal, but that that taboo was in and of itself worth tackling. If I get asked about it, I do like to point out that they don't ask if I am white when I talk about anti-racism . . .

I forgot my colleagues' names

RUTH*, FIFTIES

Night sweats and hot flushes started when I was forty-five, along with a foggy head. I'm a senior manager, and one day I was standing in reception, waiting to go to a meeting with a colleague I've known for five years. I suddenly couldn't remember her name at all. The man on reception dialled up and asked for our names. Rather than saying, 'Ruth and Ellen,' I called her 'Eleanor'. I knew there was something not quite right, but couldn't work out what.

When we got into the meeting, I saw the list of attendees and turned to her and apologized. She laughed and said she'd been a bit confused. But far better to explain than pretend it's not happening. The only reason I realized that my brain fog might be connected to the menopause is because another colleague came in one day looking very distressed and said that she was off to the GP. She thought she was getting early dementia, but in fact it was the menopause.

I am quite precise and like everything to be done one hundred per cent. I made a rare error in a budget and had a chat with my line manager. 'It's the time of life,' I said to him. Honestly, I'd rather be upfront and honest, and for there to be a medical reason, rather than him think I'm not capable of doing my job. He was absolutely fine about it.

*Name has been changed.

I left my job

SCHOOL LEADER AND BUSINESSWOMAN PAULA KENNEDY,
FIFTIES

I think that my menopausal symptoms were initially masked by having the Mirena IUS, which was taken out in 2018, when I was fifty-one. That's when I noticed that my mood was very low, and I didn't feel confident, especially at work, where I had a very senior role in a school. I felt as though I was second-guessing myself, double-checking things which I knew to be correct, and feeling a bit paranoid. That's incredibly debilitating, especially if you're dealing with staff, parents and tricky pupils while feeling as though you might burst into tears. It's hardly a professional look. Normally I'd give myself a talking to and regain my perspective, but I didn't seem to be able to do so.

I think a lot of women start to have menopausal feelings at the same time as extreme work pressure, so it's hard to separate one from the other. I knew my job was challenging, but I'd previously enjoyed that. Now, I felt that the joy had gone. If you're used to being successful and in charge, vulnerability is very hard to deal with, and I felt as though I was falling.

I spoke to friends and my partner, and after a year of this uncertainty took the decision to step down and do supply teaching, at the same time as doing a Master's in counselling, with the aim of setting up my own practice. People were very surprised; I think their perception of how I was doing the job was very different from mine! But I was too full of self-doubt to carry on.

As well as rediscovering my confidence, doing something new, and going back into the classroom and reminding myself why I entered teaching in the first place, I found my freedom. I was working very hard, but dictating my own hours to a large extent. As a vice principal, I had been doing twelve-hour days and had to be 'on' the whole time.

Now, I am working part-time again as a senior leader in the school and juggling the Master's and the mentoring programme. I am still working to set up a private practice in coaching and counselling to support school leaders, but I feel in the meantime my skills and value as a school leader are being recognized, hopefully giving me more credibility to support other school leaders in the future.

I instigated installation of fans for flushes

PROFESSOR OF SOCIAL INTERACTION, LOUGHBOROUGH UNIVERSITY, ELIZABETH STOKOE, FORTIES

Because I'm a naturally cold person, I thought that my menopause experience would be great, as I wanted to be warmer. In fact, I just looked as though someone had tipped a bottle of water over me every time I had a hot flush. I have a lot of meetings, and eventually, rather than pretend it wasn't happening, I ended up carrying around a fan I'd been given at a seminar and using it publicly. I wasn't sure what colleagues made of it! A couple of years ago, we had a new head of HR, and I suggested that we have Loughborough Purple fans available in every room. It was quite an ask in a male-dominated environment, but she made it happen and our #FansForFlushes arrived in early 2020. I posted photos, including some of my sweaty face, and was amazed that people said doing this was brave. I didn't think so, though. I just wanted to normalise something and start a more open conversation at work.

On the childless experience

MEMBER OF GATEWAY WOMEN

At my workplace, my menopause didn't coincide with any mums who were actively parenting. The difficulties I encountered were from a couple of sixty-plus mums of adult children who were 'grandmas in waiting' and seemed to assume some sort of authority as a result – they set out their stalls quite clearly about how hard (or, in their cases, not) they were willing to work. For me, menopause brought up a lot of grief, but, because that had to remain unspoken, I was in many ways expected to be a better 'team worker', i.e. more emotionally supportive (of everyone, really, not just other menopausal women) than they were expected to be to me.

CHAPTER EIGHT

Pretty Menopausal:
The Maturity Conundrum

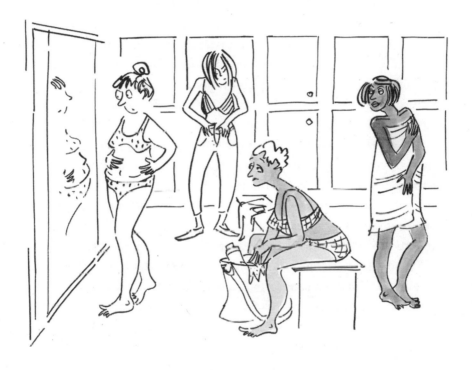

'The public changing room where you are feeling discreetly better about your flabby bits, is also one in which you can enjoy the sight of a full bush, and feel more relaxed about your grooming.'

The greatest surprise of middle age was the very first time I looked in the mirror aged around fifty and wondered where on earth my youth had gone. There I was, feeling and thinking very much like the woman I'd always been, but reflecting back at me was a shocker. Wizened. That's what I was. I appeared to have been altered by one of those instant-ageing apps that are really only funny when you're in your teens, becoming all too realistic as you speed towards higher decades! I sometimes still experience tangible shockwaves at the sight of my wrinkled face. Even with my in-head best-before date set at thirty-eight, I still shudder, imagining what my twenty-year-old self would think about what I've become!

Cruelly, the menopausal years are those during which your mental image of yourself and the physical reality start to clash, as declining oestrogen also affects face, figure and hair. Our attitudes to ageing unquestionably need revamping, but one of the heartbreaking things you discover as the years speed by is that none of us is actually prepared for the face of 'maturity', and especially not our own.

I have a theory that we all have an age at which we get mentally stuck. I'm luckier than most, because my sense of my real self, and in particular how I look, isn't fixed back in my early youth, but my late thirties, when at least there were a few wrinkles forming. Some women haven't yet reached it. Others halt prematurely, in their twenties.

This last can backfire. I'm all for women dressing exactly as they please, but whimsical florals rapidly become mumsy, and I'm not sure anyone is aiming for that. It's so easy to get stuck in a girlish groove and display, for all the world to witness, your dogged determination to keep to that path. There's a big difference between looking your best and desperately trying to look twenty years younger. Ironically, there's nothing more ageing than someone who refuses to accept their mirror image.

On the whole, I've found that base-level glamour from my late forties onwards has required both acceptance and extra maintenance. Hairs start to sprout from unusual places, such as the chin, but become less luxurious on your head. Wrinkles form that seem entirely separate from gravity, with pouchy skin forming both below and above your eyes no matter how 'clean living' you've become. Simply staying on top of the day-to-day grooming can seem an insurmountable challenge.

The question is, do you want to hop onto the aesthetic bandwagon and take your chances with every new treatment available, aiming for youth, but more likely achieving that strange Hollywood look, where you could be anything between forty and seventy? Or ought we to accept the grey hairs and wrinkles, and embrace elasticated waists as being more comfortable? Ageing is, of course, a natural process. Sometimes I worry that even plucking my eyebrows is simply succumbing to the patriarchal ideal.

In reality, I suspect that most of us settle for a happy medium, which is what I've tried to do. I have my hair done regularly, invest in pleasant face creams and had my frown line Botoxed, but otherwise I allow nature to follow its inexorable course.

You will be completely unsurprised to learn that our feelings about our looks around the time of menopause are at an all-time low, and this negativity can of course add to the overall struggle. I couldn't find many studies into women and body image in menopause; middle-aged women are the invisible sex, in many ways. But a 2014 component of the SWAN study (the Study Of Women's Health Across The Nation in the States) looked at 405 women (39.5 per cent African American; 60.5 per cent Caucasian) aged forty-eight to fifty-two and concluded that poor body image may be related to depressive symptoms.[1] Go figure!

'Women with body-image dissatisfaction were more likely to report a clinically significant level of depressive symptoms, as did women who reported feeling unattractive,' said the authors. So, if you're unhappy with your reflection and feeling pretty down about life, it is proven by actual science that it's a 'thing'. You certainly aren't alone, and you can take hope from that thought. (I'm absolutely not denigrating depression, by the way, but I don't think they necessarily needed to ask 405 women to reach this conclusion.)

Professor of Health Psychology at the University of Surrey, Jane Ogden, is fairly firm on the topic of menopausal self-loathing and looks. Firstly, she reminds us that the ageing associated with this time of life is, to some degree, inevitable. Consider the alternative: it's better to be alive and looking a bit unravelled than, well, not alive.

'You need to find your sense of identity,' she says. 'Stop being defined by how you look, and how people react to you. Yes, you may have wrinkles and age spots and your body shape has changed. But your life is written on your face and body. Lines are humour, relation-ships and struggles, which, incidentally, define you as much as happiness. Saggy bits might be from having kids or having a job which means you can't work out as much as you like. And sun damage is memories of your amazing holidays.'

The concept of wrinkles being beautiful because they are the physical story of your adventures is one with which I concur to some degree. As a travel writer and sun worshipper – contravening health, safety and fashion advice every time – I can testify to having masses of sun damage. I'd never thought of my face as a physical photo album of fun, but it's a more appealing premise than, say, 'Your complexion is your karma,' which is how I really view my multiple sunspots.

Your middle-aged skin also tells the story of your whole lifestyle, which is possibly less romcom and more psychological thriller in theme if you're low in vital vitamins and minerals and still partying like a sixteen-year-old who thinks that vodka shots and late-night fags keep you in the cool crowd. That said, the more ravaged women I know are often the most fascinating, and certainly the ones you want to hang out with past midnight, on the rare occasions you manage to stay up that late!

I know that when I drink less wine, get more fresh air, glug more water and sleep better (which often depends on how much alcohol I consume), it's all writ large on my visage. If my face is the book of my life, a couple of days of excess are a short story depicted in a pallid complexion and dark circles.

Trying too hard to keep change at arm's length is unlikely to end well, and that goes for looking after the inside as well as the outside. We've covered the practicalities of diet and exercise in chapter six, but we need to consider our thinking about food. Eating disorders among the middle-aged are on the up. 'I've been writing about eating behaviour and weight management for over thirty years,' says Jane. 'There's an increase in eating disorders among women in later life; either previous ones coming back, or new ones emerging.'

It is disheartening to discover that anorexia, bulimia and binge-eating disorders are by no means solely the remit of teenage girls. In 2012, the *International Journal of Eating Disorders* published the results of a study on eating disorders in mid-life and beyond. They found that thirteen per cent of American women aged fifty or more experienced symptoms of an eating disorder. Sixty per cent reported that their concerns about weight and shape negatively affected their lives, and seventy per cent were trying to lose weight.[2]

Jane warns that eating disorders can manifest at any time of life and are incredibly damaging. 'Eliminate vital nutrients or consume excess sugar or fat and you won't recover in the same way you might have done in your twenties and thirties,' she says. 'Plus, you put yourself in serious danger of developing all manner of health conditions' including bone loss and damage to your heart and other organs, especially during these years of hormone imbalance. Malnutrition in any form does the menopausal body and mind no favours. Quite genuinely, if you are concerned about your eating, ask for help   see your GP or contact BEAT, the eating disorders charity.'[3]

Suggesting that social media is the source of all evil doesn't count as original thought, but there's no question that a great deal of it is pretty firm on the fact that we need to remain youthful and good looking to maintain our currency. In real life, Jane says that, unless you are a model and relying on your looks for actual currency, it's unlikely that you are still going to be making friends off the back of 'being pretty'.

By the time you get to my age and beyond, people are definitely not spending time with you because you are hot and the boys want to sit at your table in the canteen. They're hanging around because you're interesting, fun, kind, hospitable, adventurous, well-informed and all the other amazing qualities that you've had a lifetime to accrue, and can keep on adding to, despite the dwindling decades in which to pursue them.

When you're young, looks are paramount because it's probably the best-looking you'll ever be, but now, happily, things even out. Those whose popularity and position depended on their superficial attractiveness often feel their value is diminished (prettiest girl in the school no more). Meanwhile, those who might have compensated for being more average find their personalities are now their greatest asset. We all get our moment in the spotlight, but some have to wait just a little bit longer to see their assets rise in value.

'Feel better about yourself by making the right comparisons,' says Jane. 'If you compare yourself to a skincare ad with an "older" but satin-smooth-skinned model who may be decades younger than you, as well as retouched, then you are going to come off badly. Compare yourself to your peer group, and you'll feel far more cheerful.' You may have a flabby tummy (nothing wrong with that, but we all beat ourselves up) but thicker hair or nicer eyes than those around you of about the same age. It's pleasantly realistic. And set your own norm. 'I didn't wear any make-up through the lockdown months of 2020,' says Jane. 'It was strange at first, but I soon got used to it. I also think it was good for my students to see me in a state of "casual-ness" so they could realize it was OK to just be themselves. Select a norm with which you are happy, not one which others are telling you to embrace, and enjoy it.'

I honestly think that there is something to relish about losing your youthful glow and not being wolf-whistled at by Neanderthals, though there's something enormously fun about looking like a younger woman from behind, with my blonde bob, and then seeing rear-view admirers recoil when they realize I'm old enough to be their mother. That famous invisibility of middle age can be dispiriting, but it's also immensely empowering.

Is it really an achievement if a stranger thinks we're hot enough to imagine having sex with? Arguably, that's what being physically admired usually comes down to. Not being noticed by men means that you can sit alone and uninterrupted in a restaurant, enjoying a good book, or have two seats to yourself on a train without some sweaty perv – first rule of perviness is that they are never attractive – trying to hit on you and ruining your alone time.

Increasingly, I find myself looking around and appreciating the diversity of beauty in age. All my friends – mostly in their forties upwards – look utterly stunning in my opinion, and young people appear rather bland and samey, not helped by the terrible trend for thick eyebrows and too much make-up, which I realize makes me sound about one million years old, and like all mothers ever. Go to any public swimming pool women's changing rooms if you want to admire the beauty in any female form, however old.

Don't stare, by the way, though there's a brilliantly confrontational scene in the TV series *The Undoing*, when Nicole Kidman's character comes face-to-face with her husband's naked and far younger mistress. Though Nicole has little to worry about on the physical front. Hollywood actresses seem to be an entirely unique species for whom normal ageing conditions, like cellulite and baby pouch, are a mystery. And they say the camera never lies . . .

I also think that this is a time during which we might have a rethink about body hair – currently, and bemusingly, unacceptable among the young. The public changing room where you are feeling discreetly better about your flabby bits, is also one in which you can enjoy the sight of a full bush, and feel more relaxed about your grooming.

Again, I'd slightly side-eye this situation, as one doesn't want to be accused of being a peeping Thomasina, but I'd certainly say that the menopausal years are ones during which we might allow our natural hair to flourish. I know the fashion for younger women is to have *montes pubis* (the Latin plural for *mons pubis*), which are as bald and smooth as eggs, and I find this a bit disturbing. But, as a friend pointed out recently, whatever your views about the aesthetics, it's not just your face that ages. I know that a million magazine articles say that it's your hands and/or your neck which reveal your true age, but I invite you to wax the hair from a fifty- or sixty-year-old vulva, and ask friends to place their bets.

It may all feel depressing, but it's society that's at fault, not us. We aren't exactly encouraged to think that we are looking our best selves. Where are all the mature women in advertising, in movies, in TV shows or media stories? We only seem to appear if we've dared to transgress what are considered the norms in terms of expected behaviour. For example, I couldn't believe the flurry of excitement generated by my innocently sharing the fact I still love a bikini, in a newspaper article, back in 2017. You'd think I'd discovered a solution for global warming, so venerated was I for a couple of days, with a multitude of 'illustrations' of my 'plucky' choice of a two-piece being dredged up, alongside equally courageous abstainers from a full swimming costume, despite bellies showing the tell-tale signs of past pregnancies.

And who hasn't felt a twinge of respect and admiration for such glorious figures as Jerry Hall, stepping out in her bathers every summer on the beach next to her house in the South of France, knowing full well that some idiot is lurking in the bushes trying to find a flaw on her sexagenarian supermodel frame so he can make a fast buck. I mean, seriously.

The problem is, if you are not being reflected back an image of yourself that gives you any confidence, it can be extremely hard to muster it when facing the world. I was so relieved to be off the dating market once I hit my fifties and the outside world confirmed what I was already feeling inside: that my value was plummeting. It may sound superficial, but I doubt it was coincidence that my long-treasured discount in designer boutiques, along with my brilliant twenty-year relationship with a top London stylist, all ended in that decade. You don't need to be a weatherman to see which way that wind was blowing!

Jane is quite right. Embracing the physical changes of menopause is about accepting a new version of yourself. I know that's easier said than done, and especially first thing in the morning when your face looks as though it needs ironing, and it takes until lunchtime for the dent from the eye mask to finally fade. But, if I've gained any wisdom at all, it's not to chase what you can't capture, and youth is something we never stop leaving behind. I very much believe that our menopausal years are those when we have a stronger sense of ourselves.

Whatever steps you decide to take towards teeth whitening, wrinkle fixing and hair colouring, don't take it too seriously, and never think that smoother skin or hiding the silver strands is the Holy Grail of contentment. Beauty does not necessarily – and I think we can all think of extremely sad beauties, both historical and current, old and young – bring happiness. Look around, particularly at real people, not magazine pages and doctored Instagram feeds, and realize that you are doing just fine – it could always be a lot worse. In a decade's time, it will be! So, enjoy the moment! You are just a new evolving version of you, and women's specialist skill is adapting to new circumstances. Don't think of it as being lesser. Just different. And, in many ways, more beautiful.

A skinful

My face has been put through the wringer over the years. Anything that I ought to have done, I've ignored, and all the basic no-nos, such as 'do not bake in direct tropical sun', I've gone ahead and embraced.

Up until the age of fifty, I felt that things were holding together quite nicely, but I noticed a definite drop in smoothness and an increase in pigmentation after that point. There's also a sort of blurring around the edges; my once firm jaw is less strong and my cheeks less defined. Some days, I look like a bad waxwork of myself, as though I have been wafted past a hot flame and melted a little.

This deterioration is for a number of reasons. Collagen is the protein responsible for skin's structure, elasticity, and that wonderful, youthful plumpness. This decreases by one per cent every year from your mid-twenties. After menopause, levels can plummet by as much as thirty per cent over the following five years, meaning that your face might sag, wrinkle and lose volume.[4]

It's been shown that the menopause may make you look older at cellular level. In 2016, an American study concluded that the cells of women who had experienced menopause speed up ageing processes by about six per cent. Great.[5]

'Alongside the falling oestrogen levels of menopause is the normal process of ageing, which is inevitable,' points out consultant dermatologist Anjali Mahto, author of *The Skincare Bible*.[6] She is in her early forties, but with the skin of a twenty-five-year-old. 'As the years go by, the skin's natural barrier function, which protects it from things going in and out, becomes less effective. This means that you lose more water. Skin also becomes more vulnerable to UV radiation and pollution, and damage from the sun adds to the mix.' These factors come together as an unpleasant group to create wrinkles, dryness, sagging and pigmentation. I'd put a tick in all of those ageing boxes, with extra menopausal effects thrown in!

What I've noticed the most is thinning skin, which occurs all over the body, and oestrogen also has a role in wound healing. Cut a menopausal woman, and she'll bleed for longer . . .

Being Caucasian, the fairness of my complexion is firmly against me when it comes to ageing. 'The darker your skin, the less rapidly you show the passing of the years,' says Anjali. 'Whilst everyone is vulnerable to the effects of chronological ageing, skin of colour often appears to age relatively slowly. This is largely down to increased pigment, or melanin, which protects against the effects of sunlight – a key factor in the ageing process.' Skin of colour also has a more compact and thicker dermis, or top layer of skin, with numerous large fibroblasts (collagen-producing cells giving support and structure), making it more resilient to wrinkling.

Studies are conflicting, she says, and little work has specifically been carried out in skin of colour. However, regardless of the menopause, it shows signs of ageing far later than white skin. 'Facial wrinkles may not develop until one's fifties or sixties, and lines around the mouth or loss of lip volume aren't common, when compared to Caucasians,' says Anjali. Thin skinned and thin lipped, that's me and my Norwegian/Irish heritage put to good use! Great. Skin of colour is, however, more prone to dryness due to a decreased level of ceramides – fats helping skin to retain moisture – compared to white skin.

In addition, our eyes look more hollow: less collagen makes them appear more sunken, and the tip of the nose may sag downwards.[7] I came across this fact by accident, but it's true. Your nose, like your boobs and your knees, may droop.

So, what solutions are there? I was hesitant about including a how-to of aesthetic treatments. I know a lot of women who have a syringe of Botox or a facial peel to look brighter and feel better. But equally, I know just as many who feel that they are quite beautiful enough and would rather go on holiday or buy a new car.

In the spirit of full confession, I've had twice-annual Botox for the deep frown lines developing between my brows, and I have also had a treatment called the Six Point Lift, conducted by a charming Frenchman called Dr Dray, which involved injecting hyaluronic acid into six points on my face. I think it assisted in the tussle with wrinkles, but no one ever commented on it, so the benefits were clearly subtle.

If you want to go down the treatment road, Anjali says that injectable treatments such as Botox and fillers are safe and provide natural results in experienced hands. 'Botox is good for tackling the development of frown or forehead lines,' she says. 'Filler can help replace the volume which is lost over time due to the thinning of facial fat. Non-invasive skin-tightening devices, such as high-intensity-frequency ultrasound or radio frequency, can also be useful for the lower face and jawline, and lasers can help improve skin texture and tone. The right treatment should be guided by an expert dermatologist or plastic surgeon, and full-face assessment should be carried out before undergoing any treatments.'

Don't be a guinea pig, don't go cheap, and don't, for goodness' sake, buy Botox on the internet and try to inject it yourself. This was a ridiculous trend a few years ago, and a browse on Google confirms that, yes, you can still do so. No good can ever come of this. You will definitely not look younger. There are forty-two muscles in the face. It would be only too easy to stick the needle into the wrong one.

What treatments you select may also depend on skin type and tone. 'The ageing process in skin of colour often starts in the middle part of the face due to changes in facial fat resulting in deepening of the nose-to-mouth lines and hollowing under the eyes,' points out Anjali. Therefore, she says that filler is often preferable to wrinkle injections such as Botox.

Another incredibly unfair potential menopause side effect is acne, which can occur even if you got through your teen years unscathed. Testosterone might become higher in relation to oestrogen, triggering outbreaks of adolescent-like spots.[8]

Rub it in

Although aesthetic treatments can be very effective, they can be flipping expensive. There are plenty of skincare basics which are appropriate for most menopausal skin types.

My mother always told me that, if you look after your face, the rest will take care of itself. Nowadays, it's clear that she was either over-optimistic . . . or lying. Nonetheless, it's advice I took to heart early on, and it's proved a habit that certainly seems to have endured. Despite many shameful debauched nights, I have never, ever, ever gone to bed with my make-up on. I'm not sure it's made any difference to my skin long term, but it certainly makes me feel smug among my girlfriends, few of whom can claim such an unblemished track record!

I'm also a sucker for good face creams, which have been my greatest investment in luxury throughout life. As I get older, I find that I need creams that are increasingly rich in texture, as my skin is definitely more Gobi Desert than lush tropical rainforest. These days, so manic is my pursuit of moisture that I top up the richest of face creams with a drop of face oil at night. I also try to avoid harmful chemicals, opt for organic products, and use night cream at any point during the day.

'When choosing good skincare ingredients to support skin health, a number of "actives" are key,' Anjali tells me. Her advice is simple: 'Nearly everyone can benefit from incorporating vitamin A and vitamin C alongside sunscreen into a daily routine.'

That's it. No miracle peptide or weird ingredients, such as nightingale poo, snail slime or human foreskin (there was a cream including this some years ago – surprisingly pleasant to use, once you got your head around the concept). No need for five-hundred-pound serums or creams created to suit your DNA. As proof – if you will – most beauty writers I know swear by this simple combination, often using inexpensive brands such as The Ordinary, Altruist and Medik8, and they all have complexions a good decade younger than their actual age. I currently follow none of Anjali's recommendations, but I am going to.

'C' ME: Anjali says, 'Vitamin C is an effective antioxidant, which means it will reduce damage caused to skin cells by harmful molecules known as free radicals. These are created in the skin by ultraviolet light from the sun, by pollution and by the body's own metabolic processes. Neutralizing the damage done can help prevent premature skin ageing.

'Use vitamin C serum after cleansing and before moisturizer or sunscreen in the morning. It's also a useful skin-brightening agent and vital for the production of collagen in the skin.'

SPF: Sunscreen should be used daily. As we've all been told countless times, you even need to apply it in the winter and on cloudy days. If you've reached or gone beyond your late forties and are already irritated by the pigmentation which flashes across your face the moment the spring sunshine starts, or have noticed wrinkles on your arms, this diktat might be making more sense.

'SPF ideally provides protection against three forms of sun damage; the well-known UVA and UVB rays, but also what's known as high-energy visible light (HEVL), which is a newly acknowledged risk. A factor of thirty to fifty is ideal,' says Anjali.

'Sunscreen use doesn't just reduce the risk of sunburn and subsequent skin-cancer development, but sunlight is the biggest factor in premature ageing of the skin. Protection will slow down the development of fine lines, wrinkles and pigmentation.'

Any part of you is subject to wrinkling. If you look at yourself in the mirror naked, you can see that the exposed bits – arms, legs, ankles, decolletage and face are all probably far more wrinkly than your thighs and boobs. Perhaps tummies and bottoms are exempt – they are under so much stress that lack of sunlight probably doesn't make that much difference.

EH, A?: Anjali says, 'Vitamin A, or retinoids, must be used at nighttime, and there is a great deal of data and studies to back up their use. Prescription tretinoin – a form of vitamin A – is the gold standard, but weaker derivatives, including the ingredients retinaldehyde and retinol, can be found in over-the-counter cosmetic products.

'Vitamin A can improve skin-cell turnover and boost collagen production, as well as target pigmentation or uneven skin tone. Sunscreen should always be used during the day, as vitamin A can make the skin sensitive to the sun.' She warns that products can be irritating to the skin on first use. 'Build up slowly and cautiously, as tolerated. Moisturizer can be applied twenty minutes later to reduce the risk of peeling or redness.'

ACNE TREATMENTS: 'We recommend the same treatment as in teenagers,' says Anjali. 'Start with topical over-the-counter products containing benzoyl peroxide, salicylic acid, niacinamide or retinol. Then there are prescription topical treatments: stronger retinoids, benzoyl peroxide or antibiotics. If there is no improvement after several weeks and spots are deep or cystic, then you may try oral medications under guidance of your GP or dermatologist – antibiotics and isotretinoin. Things usually start to settle once the menopause is over.'

Grit your teeth

Who knew that the mouth was affected by the menopause? I certainly didn't, although I am meticulous about attending hygienist and dental appointments. 'You have two key orifices which need lubrication: your vagina and your mouth,' leading dentist Dr Uchenna Okoye tells me. 'Falling oestrogen causes dryness, and, in your mouth, lower saliva flow means bacteria isn't being washed away so easily, which can lead to tooth decay and gum disease.' A lack of saliva swishing around the teeth also means that you're more likely to see staining; we all know about the potential damage from coffee, tea and red wine, but even herbal tea can give teeth a bit of a brown tinge. Nobody wants their mouth to silently scream Farrow and Ball Skimming Stone.

I have personal experience of the ageing mouth and all the joys it brings. Aged fifty, I noticed that all my lower teeth were caving inwards and went rushing off to an orthodontist, who suggested clear, fitted braces. Better than a facelift, he said, for looking youthful; teeth are vital in maintaining the structure of your face. Two years later, they certainly looked better, but then I discovered that there is no 'afterwards', and I had to add a nightly tooth retainer to my ever-expanding bedtime routine. I wonder how long I'll manage to keep up the level of maintenance. It's not the most come-hither look to be flashing a plastic tooth cover (along with eye mask and silicone ear plugs) as you settle back on the pillows of an evening, in your vintage satin.

If you are prone to the classic anxiety dream where all your teeth fall out, then stop reading now. Menopause can bring you one step closer to achieving a Tooth Fairy full house. 'The connective tissue holding teeth in place is affected by declining levels of collagen, so they may become loose, and because they're held in place by bone, post-menopause bone loss can also affect them,' says Uchenna, who also points out that I could have a fixed, permanent retainer, rather than my nightly man-repellent.

Some women also get what's called burning mouth syndrome, which isn't cosmetically displeasing, but can be quite distressing – a sort of 'burning' pain. Avoid tobacco and alcohol, she says, as well as acidic foods.

> It's not the most come-hither look to be flashing a plastic tooth cover (along with eye mask and silicone ear plugs) as you settle back on the pillows of an evening, in your vintage satin.

Uchenna sees a lot of women, around the age of menopause, who've never had any problems with their mouths, but suddenly find that things are shifting or uncomfortable. 'In your early to mid-forties, you're probably pretty complacent about your teeth if you've had a good routine for years. Then you might start noticing bleeding gums, dry mouth, twinges of pain and teeth moving around.' You may also experience such puzzling symptoms as jaw pain or a clicking jaw, which is – of course – also likely to be because of lower collagen levels. My tooth-grinding during stressful insomniac nights has actually cracked and made redundant one of my lower molars, which now has to go. My teeth also crumble and ache quite terribly. The cliché of the toothless crone draws ever closer.

The biggest problem is the fear of losing teeth – let's face it, we've all gone to the dentist months after we ought to have had an appointment, feeling sheepish and terrified. But what I find reassuring is that it's never too late to fix teeth, or their appearance, even if you do lose some. 'It perplexes me that I see a lot of women in their fifties and sixties who've suffered from problems since their forties, and are too embarrassed to see the dentist,' explains Uchenna. 'There are always solutions. People don't realize this – it's honestly rare for teeth to be beyond help, and if they are, well, I have a ninety-year-old patient who has just had an implant.' This applies to orthodontics as well; she has an eighty-seven-year-old woman wearing braces.

Lifestyle solutions include the age-old brushing and flossing, regular trips to your hygienist, and a diet high in calcium. Don't forget, says Uchenna, that kale, tofu, nuts and beans all contain good amounts of calcium. 'Avoid toothpastes containing what's called sodium lauryl sulphate (SLS). This is what makes toothpaste foam, but can also cause that burning mouth sensation.' There are some toothpastes available with extra glycerine, which can be moisturizing if you have a dry mouth. Sugar-free gum can also improve saliva flow, she says, but only chew for around ten minutes, or as long as the flavour lasts, otherwise you are pounding tooth on tooth, and that can cause more problems!

A 2017 study showed that HRT appeared to make a difference (I promise, I'm not on commission): rates of gum disease were far lower in those taking it.[9]

Heavy is the head (of hair)

My hair history is a saga in itself: three early decades of trauma, followed by twenty years during which time my glossy blonde bob was frequently described as my 'trademark'. It's always a bit disappointing to hear that any thought or idea which I've spoken over nearly six decades is nothing compared to the effect achieved by two hours in the Mayfair salon which I visited from my mid-thirties to mid-fifties.

I became entirely dependent on good hair, with any presenting job or public appearance reliant on whether or not I could squeeze in a blow-dry there. As I passed the mid-forties mark, I noticed that well-groomed hair was the perfect foil for a host of other 'imperfections' – tired skin or dark circles under the eyes, for example – and it became the number-one priority of my beauty regime.

I have always had fine hair, as well as zero skills with beauty tools, whether attempting a blow-dry or DIY manicure. In unkempt youth, hair which looks as though you've just crawled from a busy tussle between the sheets is sexy. When you're in your fifties, it's not the first image you want people to conjure up. In the last decade, I've noticed that the length can't go past my jaw without looking messy.

But, my own adventures aside, it turns out that, just like the rest of the body, hair ages, and of course the menopause can have an impact.

'Some women barely notice a difference around the time of menopause, but others will see noticeable thinning, which can be incredibly distressing psychologically,' says leading trichologist Anabel Kingsley. 'Women feel that they are losing their identity and femininity.'

And hair can hugely affect mood. A Dr Marianne LaFrance at Yale University has worked with Pantene for two decades and, in 2017, a global study by her concluded that a great hair day makes women feel strong, and was also associated with feeling 'more productive, less stressed, more socially powerful, more resilient, physically stronger and more in control.'[10] That's a lot of pressure on our hair!

'The women who come to see me at menopause feel that their identity is being challenged in a number of ways,' agrees Anabel.

There are two reasons why hair may become a concern at this time of life. Firstly, the normal growth phase of hair lasts between three and seven years, and this is maintained by oestrogen. 'A big drop in oestrogen around menopause shortens the growth phase and leads to more shedding of hair.' We all lose around eighty to one hundred hairs every single day, but, around the age of fifty, many women notice increased hair loss and seek help. This is likely to return to the normal eighty to one hundred per day range.

In addition, as oestrogen goes down, testosterone can become more dominant. Many of us have hair follicles – the bulb in the scalp from which the hair grows – which are sensitive to testosterone levels. 'In those with a genetic predisposition, follicles may become smaller and hair won't be as long or thick, with a shorter growth cycle.

'This is what's known as androgenetic alopecia, or female pattern hair loss, and is very common among women. Where men go bald, women usually see a more diffuse thinning around the head and parting,' says Anabel. It's a gradual process, and you will probably lose around twenty per cent of the density before noticing. It is said to affect up to forty per cent of women by the age of fifty – Anabel thinks that most women experience a little thinning during these years. 'There are other subtle differences. Hair becomes finer as scalp and hair-cell quality ages along with the rest of the body. Do not panic. You may not even notice.'[11]

'It's a good idea to seek help as soon as you notice thinning hair,' says Anabel. 'A good trichologist can promise maintenance of density and can often improve severe thinning, but it's not always possible to completely restore.' You can obtain prescription scalp drops containing both minoxidil and estradiol benzoate – which is topical oestrogen. HRT – replenishing oestrogen levels – can certainly help as well.

'We have a lot of clients who have had breast cancer, and always write to their oncologist to check.' You might also try minoxidil (which you can buy over the counter as Regaine for Women) on its own, which is the hair-growth scalp treatment with FDA approval (basically the gold star tried-and-tested), and is the most effective hair-growth formula for women. The only problem with minoxidil is that you have to keep using it.

Low iron and ferritin levels are often associated with thinning hair. If periods are lighter or have stopped, then this is less likely to be a problem, but if you are one of those whose periods have become far heavier, then remember that the last part of your body to receive vital nourishment is always your hair, and this is why fad diets are likely to affect hair growth.

Every hair follicle has a vitamin D receptor, so low levels can affect hair health. Anabel sees a lot of vitamin D deficiency, and especially in those of us over forty who are – too late for me – aware of sun damage.

It's easier said than done, especially if every day is a bad hair day, but try to keep stress levels down. As Anabel explains: 'Stress raises testosterone levels and creates imbalance, as well as impacting your scalp's microflora and how your gut absorbs vital nutrients, which can create problems for the hair and scalp.'

Colour Me Radiant

As for my hair colour, which has defined me for much of my career, these days it's even more fake than ever! For historical context, I developed my own badger's white stripe across my parting almost overnight, at the age of fifteen, when my father died. Back then, it was mortifying to have this blast of white hair in what I recall as being a basic mousy brown. Besides, it was the 1970s, and thanks to the original Blondie herself, and also Sid Vicious of the Sex Pistols, bleach blonde was all the rage, the less realistic the better. I've been dyeing mine lighter ever since. It's been so long that I can't truly remember the original colour, though, when I look at my daughter's tumbling locks of honey-coated gorgeousness, I know the hues didn't come from me. Now, I suspect if I let it grow out it would be pure white, which I'm thinking is the way to go to celebrate my sixtieth. Then again, they do say that blondes have more fun, and as you get older you don't want to short-change yourself on any such promises. I might hang on in there.

As if in answer to my ponderings, Josh Wood, world-leading celebrity colourist, whose clients include Kylie Minogue and Elle Macpherson, says that you don't have to do a drastic overhaul. 'As you age, and skin colour changes, think of your hairline as being a frame for your face. The colour around here needs to be a little softer and lighter, no matter what your hair type. It's all about complementing skin tone.

'Colour is a great way to make hair look thicker, especially around the parting,' he adds. 'Loss of pigment means that the scalp can be more evident; it's more apparent in darker hair.'

Colour can also create the illusion of thicker hair all over the head. 'The more contrast between light and dark, the more you give the illusion of thickness. You need to keep it multi-dimensional, with lots of different colour strands, and using techniques such as highlights, balayage and root tints.'

For those of you who like a semi-permanent colour, increased scalp sweating might mean considering permanent colour, and if you have any dye touching the scalp, have a patch test every time. 'For some reason, this is a time when you may suddenly develop an allergy or an irritation to certain products, and this can cause breakouts around the nape of the neck.'

Make-up

There was a watershed moment in my early fifties when I realized that make-up had become compulsory, unless I was in strict home hibernation. Being bare-faced no longer suggested fresh and healthy, but had become Victorian late-stage consumption. Plenty of women still look amazing and I'm consumed with envy for their natural beauty. My problem was that I'd started to lose my eyes, and, with my lopsided, asymmetrical face, that was a problem. They'd always been the feature I'd zoomed in on (long before actual Zoom, of course), but now, without a little accentuation, they just disappeared into my face. First thing in the morning, my make-up-free face is as flat and as dull as a cloudy November morning. Menopausal Ringwraith, if you like!

So, the luxury of greeting the world fully make-up free is no more a possibility for me. To mitigate, I never leave the house without a bit of Mac Omega (a lovely caramel) eyeshadow on my lids, and I have a semi-regular dedication to dyed eyebrows and lashes, which lifts my whole face. I love the Benefit Benetint Lip and Cheek Stain, which gives your cheeks that soft flush of youthful excitement – this needs faking, these days, and Trinny's BFF Skin Perfector covers imperfections and adds a fresh glow.

> Being bare-faced no longer suggested fresh and healthy, but had become Victorian late-stage consumption.

I can see exactly why make-up artist Charlotte Tilbury has become so phenomenally successful. Everything she produces creates luminosity, and that's in short supply over the age of fifty, even with a Gwyneth Paltrow-level healthy lifestyle. And, if you can buy it from Tilbury, why suffer the deprivations needed for superhuman health obsessions!

It transpires that I am neither unique nor alone with my mysteriously disappearing features. 'From about fifty-five, there's a noticeable fading of features on the face, and the paler the skin, the more evident this is,' says Tricia Cusden, the trailblazing beauty vlogger who founded make-up brand Look Fabulous Forever out of frustration at the lack of advice and make-up for older women. Her YouTube tutorials have received well over five million views.

'We call this the loss of luminance of contrast. In a younger face, you can clearly see the definition of eyes, lips, cheeks and eyebrows. But post-menopause it's not so obvious. The great thing about make-up is that you can use it to restore both colour and definition.'

I can confirm that I have lost my luminance of contrast, and am happy to take more tips on board, so I asked make-up artist Joyce Connor for advice. Incidentally, the look I think we're all trying to avoid, but one which we risk as near sight gets worse, is that slightly insane-looking caked-on look (for worst-case scenario, see Dirk Bogarde in the classic *Death in Venice* movie), with lipstick seeping into the lines around our mouths and wonky black eyeliner.

'Ideally, change your foundation every decade,' says Joyce. 'You can't keep using the same tones and textures throughout your life. As you age, I recommend using lighter-weight products such as BB creams or tinted moisturizers, and aim for warmer tones: peach or yellow (though never orange) on pale skin, and then warm up the look with a dusting of bronzer and blusher.

'Choose foundation by skin colour and undertone. A good rule of thumb is to look at veins. If your veins are blue, then you have cool undertones; aim for pinker shades. If they're green, you have warm undertones; look at shades with a hint of yellows, or reds – if skin is darker. If they're a mix of colours, then you are neutral, and might best suit beige or peach foundation. Match closely to skin colour, but err on the side of a notch darker, to create warmth. Very dark skin tones may look bluer to the naked eye and cooler tones will be more suitable. Opt for red foundation bases. And don't be afraid to change brands.'

Facial hair is an issue for many of us, she reminds me. And don't I know it. Whoever warned us that, at a certain age (particularly with an excess of testosterone gel), we'd be seeking out full facial waxing?! You can minimize the appearance of facial hair. 'Use finely milled powders and apply them with a large, fluffy-headed brush, working downwards, so the powder doesn't get under the hairs and fill them out. You only need apply powder to your T-zone and then brush it outwards.'

Primers come into their own on older skin; they are excellent for blurring, and you can wear them under foundation. 'Don't forget that, the older you are, the more concealer you need.' So true – especially in those dark hollows in the inner corners of my eyes. 'Don't apply concealer directly to wrinkles. Feather it towards them and remember you're trying to get rid of shadows, so it needs to be a shade or two lighter than your skin tone.'

> Whoever warned us that, at a certain age (particularly with an excess of testosterone gel), we'd be seeking out full facial waxing?!

'A big problem for darker skin isn't wrinkles or fading, but pigmentation,' says Joyce. 'I always tell clients to correct pigmentation using a cream corrector, then apply colour with foundation, then a liquid concealer. I call these the three Cs.'

And, for pale skin, she recommends ditching black eyeliners and mascaras. 'Black looks very harsh. Try browns, greys and navys.' Choose cream eyeshadows that swipe on and stay put. 'Glitter may look lovely, but be aware that it will sit in fine lines and wrinkles.'

As eyes start to droop, open them up by avoiding darker colours, and use a finer eyeliner. Always have eyebrows shaped to frame the eye, and tinted, if necessary, to give definition and the illusion of lifting the eye. It's a lifelong surprise to me that a well-tended eyebrow can make you look well-groomed.

Even lips shrink as you age, which I've noticed with sadness. 'Frosted and pale lipsticks risk making them look thinner, though obviously wear whatever you feel suits you,' Joyce tells me. 'Darker colours with a creamy texture will give the illusion of natural plumpness, and outline them first with a pencil.'

Cool Make-Up/Hot Flushes

Joyce says, 'To help maintain make-up all day, apply primer and then a tiny dusting of powder around your T-zone, followed by foundation. You want any oil to be absorbed to stop foundation from slipping down your face.

'If you're suffering from a hot flush, which is something I'm experiencing a great deal now, don't touch your face. Allow it to heat up and cool down, and your make-up will settle back to where it was. Afterwards, just let it dry completely, then possibly use blotting paper to soak up any remaining moisture.'

Embrace the grey

EVENTS MANAGER JESS HYDE, FIFTIES

We are menopausal women, and that's the end of it, and now I've reached my fifties, I am far more confident in who I am. In 2020, I decided to stop dying my hair and go grey. There were many reasons: I'm not organized enough to go to a salon every six weeks, I try to avoid chemicals as much as possible, and the grey hair was coming through very quickly anyway. Finally, I'm not trying to hide the fact that I'm a middle-aged woman. I lost a lot of weight in my late forties to pre-empt any menopausal weight gain, and that made me look and feel younger and – more importantly – healthier, though I'm disappointed that my tummy just shrank, rather than becoming washboard flat. I grew my hair out during the lockdown of summer 2020, and by the end of August there was enough grey that it was a statement rather than unkempt! I've had lots of compliments and absolutely no regrets. What's the point in chasing lost youth?

Burning mouth threw me for six

RESTAURANT OWNER HARRIET CAMPINA, FORTIES, ALGARVE, PORTUGAL

My perimenopausal symptoms started when I was forty-two, with terrible anxiety, hypochondria and OCD tendencies. Aged forty-six, a couple of years ago, I realized that my tongue felt as though I'd drunk a very hot cup of tea. The constant burning sensation persisted, and my mouth felt sensitive to hot things all day. It carried on for a few days, and I started to feel a bit perplexed. Then I saw a friend in her fifties. 'That's a menopause symptom,' she said. I instantly relaxed, and, a day or so later, the feeling went. It still comes back very randomly for a day or so, and it's far worse when I'm dehydrated.

Self-belief is more important than wrinkle counting

FASHION CONSULTANT NORS GOODWIN, FORTIES

This is the age at which I realize how shaped we are by our families. My mother didn't take medication or tablets, because she felt that you could eat your way through most problems. And she has the confidence of a supermodel. She walks into sari shops, this little five-foot-five lady in her seventies, and in her head she's like Elle Macpherson.

That is the attitude I'm taking into my menopausal years. Yes, you become less attractive, and people aren't looking at you, but I think we all need to recognize that there's a beauty and an honesty to ageing and getting past the stage of trying to impress. I'm hoping to get through menopause with all the exercise I do. No hot flush is going to measure up to the amount of cardio I achieve, although I have noticed I'm starting to feel warm at night! I'm not going to give up on fashion, but do what I've always done: find designers I like and buy investment pieces. I won't dress like a twenty-year-old, but equally I've no intention of going granny. Hopefully, I'll pass on my mother's confidence and self-belief to my daughters.

Susannah Constantine

WRITER SUSANNAH CONSTANTINE, FIFTIES

I lost all my confidence and self-esteem in my early fifties. The icing on the cake came when I did a shoot for *You* magazine for the publication of my first novel. It was a bit of a lifelong ambition, and I should have felt amazing. Instead, I looked at the pics, and just thought, 'Who *is* this woman?' I was frumpy and middle-aged, I'd let myself go, and was the sort of woman that Trinny and I used to help in our programme *What Not To Wear*. It was either a question of giving in and saying, 'OK, I've had my time, don't worry, it's not about how I look.' Or, I had to give it the finger and decide not to be defined by a number.

So I chose to fight ageing, but, rather than having treatments, I did it physically. I've always loved running, and I did that a lot more. I competed in *Strictly Come Dancing*, and I've taken up cold-water swimming. Slowly, I started to regain my confidence.

Now, I look in the mirror and see someone who has had a full life. It's not about looks, it's about feeling fit and well, bounding up the stairs without being out of breath, or getting up and it not taking an hour for your body to unfurl. I look at my wrinkles and I accept them. I think, as older women, we want to stand out as individuals. I can run 16 km, swim in the sea in winter and am about to go to the Outer Hebrides for two weeks, on my own, with no electricity, to write my next novel. I challenge myself. I'm grateful that shoot gave me a kick up the arse. I didn't lose my motivation. I found it, and now I project joy and self-confidence and happiness. That's far more appealing. It doesn't matter what the fuck you look like. If you're confident then people are drawn to you. Look at Copacabana beach. Everyone wears tiny thong bikinis no matter how old or wobbly they are. And they all look gorgeous.

CHAPTER NINE

The Hell of
Hormonal Insomnia

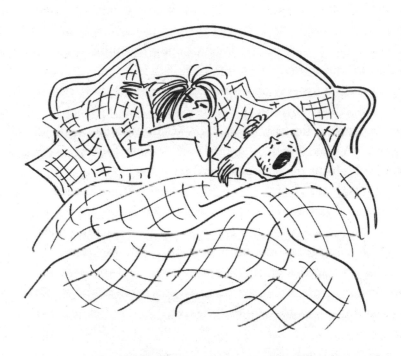

'There's no reason for us both to be deprived,
tempting as it is to nudge him awake sometimes . . .'

The other day, at a friend's house, with just the two of us there, she whispered to me, 'I think I've got that thing that you have.' I looked at her perplexed, mainly because we were alone in her kitchen, yet she was whispering. 'You know, the thing . . . that sleeping thing.' It turned out she was suffering from insomnia, but what she really meant was, 'I think I may be perimenopausal.' Menopause and lack of sleep are as closely intertwined as a pair of young lovers. There, of course, any similarity very much ends.

Personally, I love my bed. Most days, I can't get there soon enough. I sink into a deep, virtually dream-free sleep, waking bright-eyed each morning, feeling healthy, energetic and enthusiastic about the challenges of the day ahead. The night is my refuge and blissful darkness is where I retreat to regenerate and refresh.

Ha! If only. In reality, I love being horizontal between my linen sheets, and I fall asleep reasonably swiftly. But by three a.m. I am usually wide awake. Most nights I know this because I've checked the clock three times since I first crept to the loo at one forty-five a.m. Within minutes of my return to bed, I feel the delicious fog of slumber evaporate, my heart rate rise and my brain begin its relentless scan for topics to keep me engaged.

> Menopause and lack of sleep are as closely intertwined as a pair of young lovers. There, of course, any similarity very much ends.

Occasionally, I am able to raise an exhausted smile out of what I dream up as a priority worry, but more often I'm shocked by the banality of some of my thoughts. A thank-you note I failed to send a year ago, the bit part for a kitchen appliance I keep forgetting to order, how to take revenge on the patronizing BBC manager who cancelled my podcast, the name of the hedge-fund guy who might sponsor my next one, whether I booked Ocado for Friday, whether Stormzy will agree to talk to me about his favourite books, the shirt my son needs, guilt because I didn't call my friend with breast cancer, where to go on summer holidays, how to get the car to its service in Yeovil, why the woman with whom I discussed documentary ideas hasn't replied yet, did I book a blow-dry slot on Tuesday, where's that blue dress gone . . . will the world end in my children's lifetime, should I give up wine, how will we live post-pandemic?

I look again at the clock, it's three-fifteen a.m. and I'm getting closer to the moment when I'm going to either have to medicate or resign myself to staying awake. Instead, I add to my copious preoccupations: what do I have to do in the morning, and can I afford to be exhausted or should I resort to the cornucopia of drugs and sleep aids crammed into my bedside drawer for just this eventuality?

The only upside to this nightly game of insomnia roulette is that I am not alone, and I don't mean the company of a noisy bed mate, though I have that too! More than fifty per cent of women think their sleep quality is bad or very bad, according to a 2019 survey in the *Sunday Times*.[1] The same survey said that a woman who sleeps badly will average five hours, eighteen minutes a night. Welcome to the club. Serving my argument entirely, an extraordinary sixty per cent of forty-five to fifty-four year olds and sixty-five per cent of those aged between fifty-five and sixty-four said their sleep was rubbish. Coincidence? I think not. This seems to confirm poor sleep as a symptom of menopause, from peri- to post-, less well recognized but just as ubiquitous as the hot flush. That said, it's a small comfort that there are thousands of us tossing and turning furiously. Misery doesn't love company that much.

We've included an entire chapter on sleep because I am obsessed with it. Not having had enough for well over a decade, whenever I'm fortunate enough to be dreaming, I dream about sleeping. Starting the day exhausted, anticipating only your return to bed, can take a stimulating timetable from challenging and fun to flat-out horrendous. Going to the office loo and closing your eyes for a few seconds is a hiding to nothing. There's nothing so thankless as trying simply to get through the hours until you can fall into your bed that night. I have been known to make my bed in the morning and whisper, 'I'll see you later, my darling.' Something I less frequently feel the compulsion to say to my husband or children.

In 2020, I wrote an investigation for the *Observer Magazine* into what seemed to be an epidemic of sleeplessness, which appeared to affect women the most severely. Nothing I uncovered in the process diminished my conviction that women in mid-life struggle with one condition more than almost anything else: a lack of decent, restorative, regular sleep. And menopausal women top that list.

Insomnia was actually the first symptom of hormonal change that affected me, starting with baffling and frustrating nights of jerking awake and not managing to fall asleep again. I've now had poor sleeping patterns for nearly a decade, and suffered top-to-toe restlessness, from mind to legs. Fortunately, my husband falls into a snoring sort of coma at around midnight and doesn't move for a good eight hours. It's infuriating, but I suppose at least I'm not disturbing him with my tossing and turning. There's no reason for us both to be deprived, tempting as it is to nudge him awake sometimes, just so he can plunge into my nightmare for a two a.m. swim.

It's long been an expectation of later years that we sleep less. Just how debilitating and bad for us lack of sleep can be has only recently come to light. The most important thing about sleep isn't just how the next day feels, but how vital it is for our ongoing health. Not sleeping is linked to poor brain function, low mood, tiredness (obviously) and stress.

More ominously, long-term lack of sleep has links to heart disease, type 2 diabetes, respiratory problems, dementia and obesity. It's generally recognized that we need around eight hours a night, though there's no standard; between six and nine hours is enough for most adults. Those who sleep fewer than six hours a night on average have a thirteen per cent higher mortality risk than those sleeping at least seven hours. So, not sleeping properly is actually risking my health and my *life*. I dance a slow dance with Death every single night.[2]

Turn up the heat: how hormones destroy sleep

So what's keeping us awake during our peri- and post-menopausal years? Of course there are worries about children and parents, partners and careers, but far more universal than our subjective subconscious are our fluctuating hormones. Oestrogen, progesterone and testosterone all play a part in the quality of our slumber.

'Hormones affect women's ability to sleep throughout their lives, from the point of puberty, through pregnancy, and finally menopause,' says sleep expert Dr Neil Stanley. He says there may be a simple explanation. 'A recent paper suggested that the effect hormones have on sleep is merely because of the fluctuations in body temperature.' Whatever the merits of his observation, only a man would say 'merely' in that context.

'Disturbed nights can be a consequence of temperature changes created by hormonal disruption,' continues Neil. 'You need to lose around one degree of body temperature to sleep. Otherwise you're restless, uncomfortable and fidget. Women are hotter than men. It's as simple as that.'

Your body perceives a rise in heat as being a threat. With your eyes closed, you don't know whether the house is on fire, or if you're hot because of hormones. Therefore, our natural defence mechanism wakes us up, and, for many of us, that's the end of it. There is also the fact that we may have lower levels of progesterone, which can make you feel sleepy by increasing production of GABA, a neurotransmitter or brain chemical which helps sleep. It also makes you feel more relaxed.

Of course, in menopause, temperature increase is likely to come hand in hand with night sweats, the nocturnal version of hot flushes.

Some women are woken time and again at night with overheating. Once awake, you may need to change sheets or nightclothes, and, as sweat dries, you might feel cold. There are no positives. Once you've woken up, drenched and overheated, you might find you can't get back to sleep because of stress and anxiety, which might be related to hormonal changes, might be down to life stress and might be a combination of the two.

'Sleep is immensely complicated, and if sleep is disrupted you activate the stress response, which is fine in the short term, but long-term stress can lead to multiple problems,' explains Professor of Circadian Neuroscience at Oxford University, Russell Foster. He is also, incidentally, the man who discovered how our body clocks are regulated by light. My stress response is easily activated, I suspect, and it's not always to do with the menopause.

'We may be the only species who can override the biological drive to sleep – but stress is the result.' I have two dogs and can confirm that this is true. They can sleep absolutely anywhere and drop off simply by closing their eyes. I envy them this simplicity, although of course they don't have to worry about earning money to pay for the dog food. More confusingly, my husband, who *does* contribute to the dog food bill, appears to have the same ability.

When this stress response *is* activated, and for whatever reason, it all cascades in the wrong direction, like a game of Jenga collapsing. 'Elevated levels of cortisol – the stress hormone – suppress the immune system, which predisposes to infection and, long term, even cancer,' says Russell. 'Stress throws glucose into the circulation, leading to insulin resistance and a greater risk of type 2 diabetes. Sleep loss and stress lead to changes in the metabolic hormones ghrelin and leptin; ghrelin is the hunger hormone, and goes up when you're tired, and leptin, the satiation hormone, is reduced. The net effect is increased hunger, more calories consumed and weight gain.'

In summary, you will be fatter and more likely to get ill. 'Many of us are chronically tired and desperate to sleep, but the biological drive for sleep is being overridden by the consequences of being stressed to buggery,' he adds thoughtfully.[3]

Aching joints are also quite common throughout menopause. I

found that, however tired I was, on some nights my restless aching legs were able to counteract the exhaustion of my body, dancing an irritated little jig under the sheets.[4]

The other thing keeping us up is the need to pee. Frequent urination in the small hours is called nocturia.[5] The effects of oestrogen are vital for the health of the urethra, bladder and the pelvic-floor muscles. We discuss this in chapter ten (see page 247), but needing a pee at night is more prevalent around this time – in one study, seventy-three per cent of women aged forty-five to fifty-four needed to go at least once at night, and this can obviously affect sleep. So, if the flushes and anxiety don't get you, the poor muscle tone will.

As an aside, I have a number of older relatives who go to the loo quite a few times before leaving the house 'just in case', and I myself am no stranger to needing to pee in the middle of night or foolishly prolonging my wide-awake status by trying to 'hold on' till morning. We all learn over time that the need to dash to the loo almost always overrides the possibility of dropping off again. Such is the wisdom that comes with age.

Not being able to sleep can be utterly devastating, and a lack of sleep can – without exaggeration – ruin your quality of life and threaten your sanity.

Whether it's yoga, breathing your mind back to a state of calm or taking a hot bath with mineral salts before you go to bed, there are all kinds of ways to help ease yourself into better patterns. Incidentally, none of them involve scrolling on your smartphone in your bed. And, for me, the insurance of a pack of sleeping pills in the drawer is useful. Just knowing that, as a last resort, in advance of an important day, I can take one and crash out for six hours has been a major factor in maintaining my sanity over the course of my nocturnal disruptions.

Not just oestrogen

I think it's important to point out that the reasons for our mid-life sleep deprivation aren't down to menopausal symptoms alone. There's a tendency to attribute everything to the menopause, and especially if your main source of information is the internet. ('Sore ear lobes, madam-of-a-certain-age? A graze on your elbow? That will be your hormones.') During mid-life, or indeed any part of life, sleeplessness can be down to all sorts of factors. Menopausal symptoms are certainly one, but it seems relevant to include the other elements, because I find it reassuring to know, when I consider the ongoing and rubbish quality of my sleep a good six years after the menopause.

'Sleep quality naturally deteriorates with the ageing process,' says Neil. 'Here, unusually, women benefit. Men start to lose the slow, deep-wave sleep, which is restorative, from around the age of thirty-five, and women from fifty-five. Obviously, when women have events such as menstruation, pregnancy and menopause, it's hugely disruptive, but the underlying baseline doesn't shift. Men decline twenty years earlier.'

This is all because deep sleep is to do with memory, learning and physical growth; vital for kids, and obviously less so for adults. We only produce Human Growth Hormone (HGH) in this cycle. 'Post-thirty-five, men are biologically redundant,' says Neil. You have no idea how cheerful it makes me feel to write this sentence! When it comes down to it, humans appear complex, but we are really nothing more than the need to reproduce and continue our species.

> 'Post-thirty-five, men are biologically redundant,' says Neil. You have no idea how cheerful it makes me feel to write this sentence!

'Men can't hunt or protect any more, because our knees are hurting,' says Neil. 'We can still reproduce, but you don't need many men for that. Women are preserved by nature to both have babies and then to look after them.' He says that this means women are far more adaptive than men. 'Historically, you had to deal with new threats to children and new alpha males in the tribe; that's why women can multi task – because they have to, and men don't, as they just had to go out and find stuff to eat. Or kill enemies.'

So it's possible that you can't go back to sleep because there's no physiological need. 'It's not vitally important for the survival of the species.' It is – as an aside – worth pointing out that sleep deprivation is considered a form of torture.

Men and women also have different circadian rhythms. For example, men are more likely to want to go to bed later than women – you may recognize this from the twenty-first-century phenomenon of box-set watching. My husband is far more likely to say 'just one more episode' than I am. This is also evolutionary, deriving from the time when women went to sleep with the babies and men stayed up later to ensure there was no danger. Only then would they too go to bed. (These days, this state of defensive red alert is likely to be tempered by half a bottle of red and a couple of episodes of *The Bridge*).

'From about the age of ten, men and women start to go to bed later,' says Russell Foster. 'Men peak at about twenty-one and women at nineteen-and-a-half. Then they slowly move to an earlier and earlier time. But it's not until we're in our late fifties that men and women are getting up and going to bed at about the same time, and that's about two hours earlier than we did when we were in our late teens and early twenties. This is why asking a teenager to get up at seven a.m. is like asking a person in their late fifties to get up at five a.m.'

When men do go to bed, they often disturb the lighter (in weight) and lighter-sleeping women, who then struggle to go back to sleep. The general increase in obesity means men are more likely to snore or suffer from sleep apnoea, which is also disruptive, and especially as they get older. About forty per cent of adult men are habitual snorers, though they are less likely to snore from the age of seventy onwards. 'If you can find an alternative sleeping space, it does not reflect upon the state of your relationship. Indeed, better sleep may make you happier, healthier and even a more fun partner,' says Russell.[6]

Indeed. While I diligently attempt to follow the CBT advice I've been given and count my breaths – five in, five out – to restore my equilibrium and compartmentalise the turmoil, my husband snores deafeningly beside me, deep in a contented sleep that not even the alarm clock can halt. If he knew how close to homicide this nightly inequity of rest brings me, he wouldn't be so relaxed. I counsel myself by remembering it's not his fault, but it's certainly not helpful that so many women's attempts to get back to sleep are challenged by their noisy partners. Another compelling reason to explore any latent lesbian impulses.

'Also, on the plus side, sleep in women is designed to be relatively flexible from an evolutionary point of view,' says Neil. 'They cope. So women are more able to recover from sleep deprivation, and also to rebound better from very little sleep. At the end of the day, men are there to protect and procreate; by nightfall, their job is done.' Lucky them.

Too stressed to stop

The other reasons for poor sleep at this time of life are, as you'd expect, because of our day-to-day stresses.

Not only are we busier than ever before, but the structure of the family has changed, and this has put more onus on women. 'We've shifted from the extended family to the nuclear family within almost a generation and a half,' says Russell. 'This means that childcare is no longer the responsibility of the extended family, but focused on the parents, and especially the mother. So the mother is on call all the time and this leads to awful guilt that you're not coping. We're not evolved to be able to cope by ourselves. In all primate societies, child-care is distributed across the extended family.'

By the time you've reached menopause, this is quite likely to still be the problem. Small children are at least reasonably static, but, the more they grow, the more they want to visit places. As the mother of two teenagers, I am not so much a maternal presence as an unpaid taxi service-cum-laundry woman and twenty-four-hour buffet provider, and I do this as well as working full time. I constantly feel bad about not devoting enough time to them, not that they'd necessarily want me around more, incidentally.

This is also an age at which parents may need more support. I have many friends who are in the position of being at least a part-time carer – not in any way grudgingly. Childless menopausal women (whether by choice or not) point out that they are often expected to do more with elderly relatives or at work because of their perceived lack of commitments. For those who wanted but didn't or couldn't have children, this may painfully coincide with their grief that fertility has come to a finite conclusion.

A member of Gateway Women says, 'Now I am menopausal and struggling with getting enough sleep at night – hot flushes mean some days I feel completely exhausted and I don't want to work ridiculously long days to cover others' absences. Any time off I get for working long hours I usually spend alone, as the majority of my friends have children/grandchildren and are engrossed in being matriarchs with other matriarchs.'

Our guilt or overwork translates to stress and therefore sleepless-ness and, in some women, depression. 'We know one of the destabil-izing effects of sleep on physiology is that it increases the chances of being in a depressive state. Once sleep starts to slide, your physiology goes, your sleep gets worse and the stress increases. The first sign of depression is a changed pattern of sleep,' points out Russell.

> As the mother of two teenagers, I am not so much a maternal presence as an unpaid taxi service-cum-laundry woman and twenty-four-hour buffet provider, and I do this as well as working full time.

Think of all the distractions that surround us, as though we needed any other reason to stay awake. In the past, you put the last lump of coal on the fire and then went to bed. Now, we have 24/7 everything: telly, shopping, emails, social media and work. Our evolutionary adaptation can't keep up with technology. Humanity, and especially women, have more to distract them from sleep than ever. In fact, in 2017, Netflix CEO Reed Hastings claimed that the streaming giant's biggest rival is our need for sleep. 'You know, think about it, when you watch a show from Netflix and you get addicted to it, you stay up late at night,' he said. It's designed for binge watching. That's why there are only a few seconds between episodes.[7]

'Our individual sleep patterns are like shoe size,' says Russell. 'One size does not fit all; some people need nine hours and others only need six. The key thing is to work out if you are a long or short sleeper and then try and defend your individual sleep needs.'

We fret about waking up, but some of us don't automatically sleep through the night in one swoosh of eight hours. Instead, we might wake up once or a few times, and some of us may stay awake for a while.

Calling a halt: the solutions

The ridiculously long list of medications and supplements in my armoury rather proves that there's no simple solution. I take my daily HRT, in the form of oestrogen gel in the morning and a progesterone tablet in the evening. I assume this helps – I have no intention of exploring the landscape of an HRT-free life. As we've said, HRT is great, but it's not a cure-all. And it doesn't quite tick the sleep box for me.

I've also tried CBT breath counting (it works, but some nights it proves impossible to stop the thoughts flooding in), CBD oil (quite helpful), having a bath with lavender oil (occasionally helpful), sleeping pills (very helpful, but I don't want to be addicted), white noise (better than just the sound of my thoughts rattling around), melatonin (in small doses, and taken regularly, it definitely helps, and it's available on the NHS for over-fifty-fives), Horlicks (just makes me thirsty), doing less work (works a treat, but hard to pay the bills) and the Calm app (again, better than my own thoughts, but often they break through the rippling watery noises and scare me). Magnesium – oral or topical – is good for aching and restless legs, and, fortunately, I enjoy reading, which doesn't send me off to sleep, but helps me while away the small hours.

Professor Kevin Morgan at Loughborough University is also a sleep expert, and he – bafflingly – doesn't necessarily recommend my scattergun approach. 'Most women will experience some sleep disturbance during menopause,' he says. 'It introduces a range of unique but ultimately predictable challenges to sleep, which will be – hopefully – short-lived for many. Very few women emerge from those years with permanently disturbed sleep – but some will.

'The problem with, say, sleeping tablets or melatonin is that they offer only short-term solutions for what can be a longer-term sleep problem,' he says. 'If you address sleep problems with a pharmacological response, it pays to consider your exit strategy, since you may be committing yourself to a product for the rest of your life.'

It's a valid point, but perhaps made by someone who doesn't seem to have experienced the agonies of permanent exhaustion. Just a few years of insomnia can feel like a life sentence and culminate in ruined careers, relationships and quality of life.

Treat sleep

HRT
This has been shown to help reduce night sweats, which are the whispering fiery demons of the menopausal woman's night. Progesterone also helps you to relax and is known to increase the production of a brain chemical called GABA. Low testosterone can also affect sleep.[8]

Sleep Clean
Apologies for repeating this sleep hygiene advice, which seems terribly obvious. But it makes a huge difference to have a bedroom

that meets your needs. Experts are quite correct when they recommend that your room be as cool as possible and that you wear natural fibres to wick away moisture, as well as using cotton sheets. 'If you get hot and sweat stays on the skin, sweat evaporation is switched off, and you get hotter,' points out Neil.

Don't do anything before bed to increase body temperature: eating late, drinking too much alcohol or doing vigorous exercise, although exercise during the day does help sleep quality. And we all know about leaving gadgets downstairs.

'Another – controversial – suggestion is not sleeping with your partner,' says Neil. 'They can be like a big hot water bottle, and many women lie in bed suffering rather than disturbing their partners, such as by opening a window.' Clearly, this can come with its own downsides.

Get up and go to bed at the same time every day. This maintains your body clock.[9]

Bitter Pill? Melatonin

'Melatonin isn't a sleep hormone,' says Russell Foster. 'It's a biological marker of the dark and it modulates but does not drive sleep.' As the day turns to night, the body produces melatonin, as one of many signals that it's time to go to bed. People with heart problems, on beta blockers and the elderly have lower levels of melatonin, and this may contribute to the poorer sleep seen in these groups of individuals. As a supplement, it's been used for slightly inducing sleepiness, and is only available on prescription in the UK in the over-fifty-fives.

'Part of the problem is that sometimes melatonin works and sometimes it doesn't,' says Russell. 'Some people seem to be quite sensitive to it and some aren't. All the evidence suggests that it isn't dangerous. The only thing I'd be careful about is if there is a family history of mental illness, as there is some evidence that it might lower mood.'

Working it Out: CBT

'It's the frontline treatment for insomnia,' Neil says, and it's supported by the NHS, the EU and the US. He says it's as good as, if not more effective than sleeping tablets. 'Whatever CBT process you choose, and you can pay potentially hundreds of pounds for courses, remember that they all have the same components. It's like making a Victoria sponge. There are the same ingredients, but delivered in different ways.'

CBT (also see chapter five, page 126) is about reframing the fact that poor sleep is just a bad habit, and learning what affects sleep. Free on the NHS is Sleepstation.org.uk (though you have to get a GP referral, otherwise it costs), and another site, Sleepful.me, with lead author Kevin Morgan and run by the National Centre for Sport and Exercise Medicine, Loughborough University, is also free to use. 'We used public money, so we rather felt we'd like to give something back,' says Kevin. Words which I'd love to hear from any government ministers claiming extraordinary expenses.

> 'We used public money, so we rather felt we'd like to give something back,' says Kevin. Words which I'd love to hear from any government ministers claiming extraordinary expenses.

Naturally Tired: Supplements

There is some evidence of efficacy for valerian, passiflora and hops. Passiflora is said to reduce brain activity and help sleep. Valerian has sedative effects, but nobody seems quite sure why – though it's thought it might be related to GABA production as well. And hops also appear to affect melatonin and the happy hormone serotonin.

'They've been mentioned since the fifteenth century, so purely on the basis of longevity there's certainly a belief that they work. Remember that, just because they're natural, it doesn't mean there aren't contra-indications with prescription medication. Always check,' says Neil.

I know a few people who swear by the Bach Rescue Night Remedy, which contains white chestnut, said to help switch off the mind from unwanted repetitive thoughts, but I couldn't find any conclusive clinical studies.

There is some good evidence of magnesium's usefulness (see chapter six, page 153). It helps with leg cramps and muscle relaxation, and those who have trouble sleeping often have low levels of magnesium. Magnesium and melatonin together are said to be especially effective.[10]

How Does Sleep Work?

Dr Neil Stanley

The body runs on a twenty-four-hour cycle known as the circadian rhythm. Going to bed and getting up at the same time successfully maintains this. The dark stimulates the body to release melatonin, which makes you feel sleepy.

We all sleep in cycles of around ninety minutes, each of which consists of four stages: light sleep, deeper sleep and the deepest sleep, or slow-wave sleep. The final stage is REM, our dream sleep. As the night goes on, this stage gets longer. Ideally, you wake at the end of a sleep cycle, when your body is preparing to wake up.

As we wake, the brain secretes less melatonin and higher levels of the stress hormone cortisol. At the same time, blood pressure and core temperature rise.

My life became hellish

INTERIOR DESIGNER MARIA MATTHEWS, FIFTIES

I've always slept really well, but one night, aged forty-eight, I suddenly stopped being able to drop off. I was exhausted, my eyes sleepy and heavy. But then I'd turn out the light, and instantly this strange pressure started building up in my body. My heart raced relentlessly and I felt as though my eyeballs were alive, in spite of being covered by my eyelids. I'd press on them to stop them moving. The entire night was spent feeling as though I'd just been jolted awake by the sound of a burglar, in a terrible state of fight-or-flight, lasting till dawn.

After a month, I went to the doctor. By then, I could barely function, and I almost crashed the car driving back from the school run, because my reflexes were so sluggish. I was given sleeping tablets, in the form of zopiclone, and for two years I meted them out like gulps of water in a desert, allowing myself two nights of decent sleep a week: oases of peace in between the long, frantic nights.

My husband and I ended up in separate bedrooms for a while, and I felt incredibly isolated, as well as depressed and exhausted. I was like an old woman, but without even the ability to nap during the day.

I can't express strongly enough how terrible menopausal insomnia can be. It's no exaggeration to say that it ruined my life. Now I've emerged from this in-head hell, I look back on that time with horror – as does the rest of my family.

The heat of the night sweat

BUSINESSWOMAN JANE HALLAM, FIFTIES

Apparently, during a hot sweat, you lose the same volume of perspiration as you'd lose in a forty-five-minute gym session, but in the space of two or three minutes. My night sweats started when I was forty-eight, at the same time as my sleeping stopped. I'd wake up completely drenched, literally soaked through to the skin, a few times a night; and remember, you can only move to the other side of the bed once. As I couldn't get back to sleep afterwards, I felt as though I had completely lost my mind, and found it difficult to function during the day. As soon as I slept again, the hot flushes would rear up. In the end, it's been a benefit; I designed a range of sleepwear which is comfortable for menopausal women.

Laura Collins

NHS WORKER LAURA COLLINS*, FORTIES

Bed has always been my favourite place. I've never understood people who say they have a problem sleeping. I used to get into bed, snuggle under a 15-tog duvet and drop off instantly. I could sleep anywhere: trains, planes, cars . . . Then, two years ago, it all changed. Every night, my wife Kate* and I used to chat and then spoon, falling asleep together. But not any more. Since I turned forty-five, I've been woken a minimum of five times a night with night sweats; jolting awake boiling hot and drenched and then becoming freezing cold as the sweat dries; going from one extreme to another. On a bad night, it can be fifteen times. I have become heat intolerant and I get too hot in the same position. I feel I have to distance myself, even though we're sleeping in the same bed. I think it's quite hurtful – she understands why, but is sad to lose physical closeness. She's a specialist nurse and is very sympathetic; she has to get up earlier than me in the morning, and always tries not to disturb me.

Kate* and I loved clubbing and dancing till three in the morning long after our friends settled down for early nights, but, since March 2020, I've gone to bed early, and without the same anticipation, not knowing how much sleep I'll get.

*Names have been changed.

CHAPTER TEN

Hot Sex

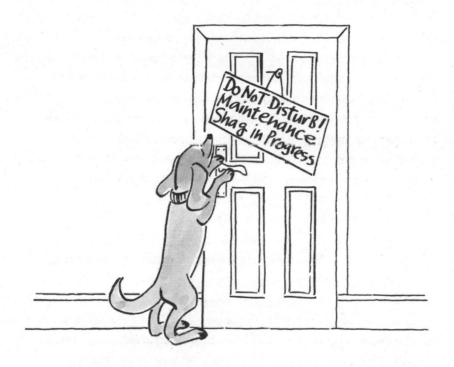

'Sex helps with low mood, by both releasing oxytocin,
a happy hormone, and reducing the stress hormone cortisol,
as well as providing a handy inner workout.'

As luck would have it, the very week I sat down to plot this chapter, the doorbell rang, and I was presented with a tasteful-looking box of what I believe are known as feminine hygiene products: pretty pastel-coloured boxes full of items specifically for the vagina and vulva. Perhaps I'm oversensitive, but there seems something vaguely judgemental about the term 'hygiene', when juxtaposed with 'vagina', as though it's a dirty place that needs scrubbing up. I am also wary of the word 'intimate', which seems irritatingly coy.

I'm not unused to unhealthy attitudes towards women's sex organs. Having grown up during those dark ages when men used to shudder at the very mention of that fishy-smelling no-go zone worthy of penetration only, it's still a pinch-me moment to find myself in an era when Gwyneth Paltrow's This Smells Like My Vagina candle is a bestseller.

One of the reasons I accepted a role in a sell-out run of *The Vagina Monologues* in 2001 (I was totally obscured by the brilliance of my two partners: actresses Marianne Jean Baptiste and Amy Irvine) was because of the subversive delight in saying the words 'vagina' and 'cunt' a hundred times a night, in celebration rather than trepidation. Image improvements aside, it's a body part that generally misses out on the self-care we give our faces, hands and feet, and, other than being the hotspot for sexual pleasure, unless we're pregnant or have an STI, it tends to barely feature in our maintenance schedule. That all needs to change in middle age, when sweet-smelling and specifically designed products are barely grazing the spot, so to speak.

It's not just the more commonly publicized difficulties that can present, like vaginal dryness, an endless propensity to pee and recurring urinary tract infections, but also thinning pubic hair and, rather upsettingly, I discovered it's not just the top of your head that goes grey! The day I found my first grey pube, I seriously considered booking my slot at Dignitas. It's a shock to the system, I can tell you, and another hurdle to surmount, to avoid falling into a muddy puddle of deep mourning for our lost youth and our poor, lustrous, gleaming pubes!

> The day I found my first grey pube, I seriously considered booking my slot at Dignitas. It's a shock to the system, I can tell you, and another hurdle to surmount, to avoid falling into a muddy puddle of deep mourning for our lost youth and our poor, lustrous, gleaming pubes!

As for nit-picking between 'vagina' and 'vulva', if I dare expose further my own ignorance, the differences between the two are something I only became aware of myself recently, such are the mysteries that surround female biology. If you Google them, I'd advise that you 'stay alert', as the government slogan during the COVID-19 pandemic suggested. It can be a fast track to the dark web, unless you're very careful!

Anyway, back to the newly delivered box. Within, I discovered an entirely new world, devoted to the most personal of beauty ranges: a Daily Intimate Wash, an Intimate Calming Oil, various other scented lovelies and a lollipop shaped like a vulva, which, having been on a sugar-free diet for two weeks, I immediately ate. I was relieved to find it wasn't cunnilingus flavoured, à la Gwyneth.

Skincare for sex organs seems yet another addition on the to-do list for a generation of women already juggling responsibilities like circus professionals, and I'm inherently suspicious of any routine devoted to wiping out my natural odour (although, if Annick Goutal did an Eau D'Hadrien 'intimate spray', I might be tempted to take my perfume lower than my neck). It's hard enough remembering to cleanse, tone and moisturize my face every day. Seriously, adding further chores isn't an option unless they're essential.

However, it appears that these just might be necessary new to-dos. The indignities do indeed seem to pile up at just the time that you're not feeling particularly well equipped to deal with further adversity. The good news is, with a little bit of concentration, an embracing of the inevitable and the determination to maintain a manageable self-care routine, it doesn't need to be the end of the world for your body below the waist! But it's certainly a bit more effort. You can't just lie back and think of England. Or, in the interests of inclusion, Scotland, Wales or Northern Ireland. Incidentally, I did test out those 'intimate' products, and they were lovely to use and wonderfully effective. I'm sure Gwynnie would approve.

The bare facts

What we aren't told about the possible state of our vaginas from our forties onwards is, I discover, quite shocking. The vagina is obviously a vital part of the reproductive system. It's important for both making babies and getting them out, as well as providing a great deal of entertainment and hospitality.

But the vagina and vulva never score top billing on lists of symptoms, always playing second fiddle to the flashier, certainly more obvious, and perhaps more palatable, hot flush. It's almost as though the general assumption is that older women shouldn't be having sex, and it's certainly not worth keeping ourselves booty-call prepared. Don't get me wrong, discussing it as frankly as I am here raises a blush, and has involved some heated internal debate, but my desire to bust the cycle of shame has overridden any sense of decorum I'd hoped to maintain.

To summarize the areas of concern: the vagina is the muscular canal with the cervix at the top. If you're heading upwards, it's where sperm travels to find the egg, and, going down, it connects the uterus to the outside world, so that babies and menstrual blood can come out. It's around three inches long, but is of course super stretchy.

The outside bit is the vulva, which includes the opening of the vagina, also known as the vestibule; the labia, which has inner and outer lips; the opening of the urethra, where the wee comes out; and the clitoris. Like the rest of the body, the vulva and vagina alter with age, and never more so than at times of hormonal flux.[1]

As we know, oestrogen controls lubrication; dry mouth and dry eyes are common as it declines. But it's also essential for the health and comfort of the bladder, vagina and vulva. Take away natural hydration, add in thinning skin, alter the pH levels, remove the muscle tone, and you're potentially facing all manner of problems.

There can be dryness, itching, soreness and pain during inter-course and urinating. The wall of the urethra, the duct which carries urine from the bladder, becomes thinner and more sensitive, the pelvic floor muscle loses tone, which can mean leaking urine, and there's an increased likelihood of urinary tract infections (UTIs) and thrush. The vagina becomes shorter, tighter and the skin less elastic.

This all comes together in a rather unspeakable phrase: genito-urinary syndrome of menopause. Makes you shiver with horror, no? It is also called vaginal atrophy (and most often Googled as vaginal dryness),[2] which is no less unpleasant in connotation, but slightly more usefully descriptive. It's thought that around eighty per cent of us suffer problems with our vaginas and vulvas during and after the menopause, and it can start as very subtle signs, such as discom-fort during a smear test, as early as your forties. There is no way of knowing how many women actually suffer, because most endure what can be genuinely torturous symptoms in silence and don't dare seek medical advice. Very few women, me included, particularly want to confide in our GPs – assuming that you can get through to them, speak to a female doctor and be considered in enough discom-fort that you're allowed to pop in for a red-faced (and possibly pants-down) experience.

Studies offer clues. In a 2013 paper called 'The Silent Epidemic',[3] the author said that most women would suffer problems with the vagina and lower urinary tract, but reported that forty-two per cent didn't seek treatment for such problems as it 'wasn't important' and thirteen per cent considered it was 'something to put up with'.

When I found myself regularly getting cystitis on the dwindling occasions my husband and I managed to squeeze intercourse onto our to-do list, I was puzzled. Surely this is a condition synonymous with carefree youthful coupling, when you'd be at it all night, and wind up suffering for your enthusiasm with the need for a bath in baking soda to ease the burning.

I had no idea that, for entirely different, and far less erotic reasons, even routine love making of swift duration could induce similar agonies; the urethra is more likely to get infected if you're lacking moisture, and also because of the thinning skin and a change in the local bacteria.

After a few months of this debilitating condition recurring, at a routine doctor's appointment I slipped it in as a seemingly inconsequential last-minute query, with my hand already on the door. Luckily, I'd asked the right person: far from increasing my evident discomfort, family GP Dr Martin Scurr advised me that, for a woman, urinating within fifteen minutes of having sex can wash away the bacteria and save menopausal mid-lifers from the all-too-common symptoms of cystitis. Other treatments include being well hydrated, using over-the-counter painkillers and – if needed – antibiotics.[4]

As my story proves, staying silent is not the answer; I subsequently only had the odd bout of cystitis, but it was a glimpse into the world of a quite extraordinary lady I came across, called Jane Lewis. She suffered from seriously debilitating vaginal atrophy for seven years, from her early forties, and wrote the compelling – I mean this, it's hilarious – book called *Me and My Menopausal Vagina*,[5] with her daughter, and she agrees.

'Women aren't seeking help for vaginal atrophy symptoms, and by not doing so are perpetuating the feelings of secrecy and shame,' she says. 'Only about seven per cent will go to their doctor, because they're so embarrassed. But if GPs don't see the condition, and how many women are suffering, then they won't get educated, and it becomes a vicious cycle.' Many medics have read her book and suggested that it needs to be on their curriculum. Vaginal atrophy can, she says, destroy your quality of life. 'It's the forgotten symptom and, quite genuinely, a sore subject.'

She describes her experience thus: 'Imagine if you had a really dry mouth, but couldn't drink anything, so it splits and cracks and bleeds and burns. You'd be aware of it every second of the day.' Jane recounts being unable even to sit down because of the burning pain, and using tins of frozen baked beans wrapped in a towel to press against her nether regions to temporarily alleviate the agony. To me, this undignified solution is reminiscent of childbirth – you get to a point where you simply don't care what happens, as long as the pain stops.

Her experience – basically seven years of well-documented suffering – is both eye opening and eye watering. In spite of having the most extraordinarily supportive family, she was in such distress that she considered taking her life. 'One day, my daughter called up and kept me on the phone for ages. I thought she was at work, but then she arrived on my doorstep. She says that she was worried I might harm myself.'

Did she have sex during this time? 'What do you think? For some women, sex becomes painful, so they stop having it entirely. Then the pain goes, but this means the area is completely unused. Pelvic exams become impossible, or you may get repeated UTIs [which chimes with my own experience], and then the whole vulva area becomes sore, itchy and burns when you wee.'

'My experience sounds dramatic, but it's certainly not rare,' she says. 'Women put up with things and self-treat, but it's not necessary.' Perhaps you are reading this and nodding a little bit, even grimacing, in recognition, and realizing that repeated UTIs is not normal, as you suspected, or that painful sex might have a solution. Have a chat with your GP, who may help or can refer you to a menopause clinic.

Two years after writing her book, Jane is – you will be relieved to hear – in a far better place, relatively speaking, but she reminds me that this is for life.

'I still can't wear skinny jeans, I'll never ride a horse again and I don't let my guard slip, but I can sit in the cinema. I have a routine: I wash twice a day with water, and I apply moisturizer. You aren't suddenly going to start producing more oestrogen. If you need local oestrogen – one of the most effective treatments (as a gel, pessary or ring) – that's going to be forever; don't be fobbed off with a short course. And don't let anyone tell you that you can't take HRT and use local oestrogen. Yes, you can.' She adds that, when you do a monthly breast check, you should include a vulva check as well.

For this, she says, you need a good hands-free mirror and good light. Sit on the bed with your legs apart and look at the vulva. 'Touch, feel, look for tears, ulcers, splits, whiteness, redness, inspect the whole outer area, then open the inner labia, or vestibule, and repeat.'

If you see anything untoward, take a photo, make notes and, if it's still there after a month, go and see your GP. 'Don't self-treat. The symptoms of VA are very similar to other skin conditions which have potentially serious consequences if left untreated, such as lichen sclerosus and vulval cancer.'

In addition to few of us being comfortable discussing our private parts, sexual difficulties can be perceived as shameful. 'It's very hard to persuade some communities, especially those with a strong faith, to chat about this subject,' says NHS GP Dr Nighat Arif. 'Sexual difficulties are likely to be blamed on the women. They worry that their husbands will take another wife.'

In the same study about how many women sought help, it was pointed out that, 'In Arab countries and the Middle East cultural and religious taboos regarding sexual life and related issues inhibit many women from discussing vaginal dryness and sexuality issues with healthcare providers.'[6] But you don't need to leave UK shores to find yourself in a culture of silence on such matters.

Nighat says that there's conflict between GP knowledge of vaginal atrophy as well. 'Excess discharge can be a symptom, but fluid suggests that there's sufficient hydration in the area, so it's dismissed as a cause of pain.'

I think that a life's work devoted to this beneath-the-bikini-line subject is time well spent. Jane even produced and paid for ten thousand leaflets about the condition to be handed out in GP surgeries, and Nighat translated it into Urdu for the Pakistani community.

Gel up

In my day, we used to snicker about K-Y Jelly, but as you reach maturity, one of the new generation of sexual lubricants without harmful chemicals (no one should be shoving anything with the potential for irritation into their most intimate parts) is not just a bottom-drawer aid to kinkier diversions, but essential for routine coupling. Yes, your bedside table needs to contain a tube of lube. But it's not that simple.

Walk into a large pharmacy and shuffling up the sex aisles offers a baffling array of products. It's a sight for all the sore parts. There's plain, there's silky, sensual, strawberry and there's sensitive. What a world. The temptation is to either swear off sex for the rest of your life, or grab the first product to hand and leg it. Visit any sex site and it's just as hard to make a decision. As I mentioned earlier in this chapter, lubrication may be the secret to post-menopausal sex for the majority of women, but which is right for me?

Strongly suspecting it might not be as straightforward as 'choose the cheapest', I asked ex-nurse Sam Evans for her thoughts. She now runs an online sex-toy retailer, and gives a great deal of advice to menopausal customers about having comfortable sex. She combines knowledge with extreme frankness – I have all sorts of, not entirely relevant, questions about vibrators – and feels very strongly about vaginal health.

'There is this myth that our vaginas need to be scrubbed, tight and fragrant. This needs to be debunked.' To this end, she says, there are an awful lot of products purporting to freshen, perfume and even deodorize the area.

> Yes, your bedside table needs to contain a tube of lube. But it's not that simple.

'Focus on cleanliness and moisturizing,' she says firmly. Avoid using perfumed products such as shower gels. Sex may be easier (or possible) when using sexual lubricants. But many ingredients might make dryness and irritation worse.

In fact, buy the wrong product and you may cause more problems than you solve. A 2018 study by the University of Guelph in Canada found that ninety-five per cent of women use feminine hygiene products such as wipes, sprays and creams at some point in their lives. But these seemed to come at some risk; those using gel sanitizers were eight times more likely to have a yeast infection and almost twenty times more likely to have a bacterial infection. Feminine washes or gels also increased the possibility of bacterial infection and urinary tract infections.[7]

Be gentle, says Sam. Scented products can be irritating, glitter is definitely not wise, and avoid chemicals such as parabens, glycols and glycerin (a sugar), which can cause thrush. 'Don't look at the colour, look at the ingredients.'

Wash your vulva and vagina with water, she says, but do not steam it. This was a huge trend a few years ago, and advocated by all manner of A-listers. The theory is that it's super cleansing. The reality is more likely to be third-degree burns, and heating the area may increase the risk of bacterial or yeast infection.

And don't over-cleanse. 'As well as potentially adding to the distress of existing problems by using items containing the incorrect ingredients, it's really important to ensure that you maintain good bacteria levels around the area,' points out Sam. 'These exist to protect the vagina and vulva, and you're more likely to develop infection by maintaining obsessive hygiene levels.' A good vaginal moisturizer, again free from irritating ingredients, can make a huge difference to sexual health and pleasure.

Incidentally, bring up the subject of a well-tended vulva and be prepared for controversy. The porn star 'ideal' is sexist and wrong, but Alexia Inge, founder of beauty website cultbeauty.co.uk, launched a female pleasure and wellness section in 2018. This includes vibrators, lubes, pelvic-floor trainers and vaginal cleansing products. '#MeToo exploded that traditional, po-faced reaction about women's sexuality, and meant that we could speak more freely about the subject,' she says. 'At the end of the day, the vagina is just a part of the anatomy.' But the reactions on social media made her reel. 'We asked an artist to do cut-out paper vulvas, and had women arguing on all channels over whether our children ought to see such images (in a world of easily accessible porn), and "How dare we say vulvas need to be clean"!' She says they've never seen such a reaction to any product launch.

Buzzing off

How is it not common knowledge that regular orgasms are more than just a fun pursuit? For a start, they can help with poor sleep – releasing a hormone called prolactin, which makes you feel relaxed.[8] Sex helps with low mood, by both releasing oxytocin, a happy hormone, and reducing the stress hormone cortisol, as well as providing a handy inner workout.

Vibrators, or sex tech, are not just a racy add-on to youthful sex, but another must-have bedside drawer companion for middle-aged women. I have one friend who keeps her 'Bullet' – a lovely little lipstick-shaped vibrator – in her handbag, in case the opportunity arises for a quickie in a loo cubicle during the working day. Is it coincidence that she has never struggled with her sex life and she's now sixty-two? I think not.

> I have one friend who keeps her 'Bullet' – a lovely little lipstick-shaped vibrator – in her handbag, in case the opportunity arises for a quickie in a loo cubicle during the working day.

You wouldn't think that our menopausal years would necessarily go hand in hand with experimental eroticism, but I really don't see why not. If penetration is painful, then work around it. I don't think I need to explain in too much detail, but I do like the word 'outercourse', which is nice and descriptive. In my early fifties, I spent six months compiling an anthology of erotica called *Desire*,[9] and I can assure you my purpose was in equal measure selfish and magnanimous. It was also a glorious and sensual reawakening, during which time it was hard to entice me from my 'research'.

On a more pragmatic level, you need to keep the vagina busy to keep it supple and lubricated. Sam recommends that women use small, slim vibrators to help open and tone the vagina (you can buy 'dilator' kits, like Russian-doll vibrators, which get gradually larger), should you be post-menopausal and not sexually active (or in a long-term relationship, would be my addition). Ensure you always buy vibrators covered with 'skin safe' silicone or made from metal, plastic or glass, which are non-porous and easy to clean. Avoid jelly, latex and rubber, and make sure you buy from reputable retailers. There are – she says – fake, stolen and used products sold online! I've heard single friends joking about their 'virginity growing back' after a few months of no sex. In some ways, this is sort of the case – the fact is that the more you 'use' your vagina, whether it's through sex or vibrators, the better.

You certainly don't have to have a partner. Female masturbation is one of those taboo subjects, historically seen as either repulsive, dangerous to our delicate kitten psyches (and, in Victorian times, could mean you got popped in an asylum if you were unlucky) or the stuff of male fantasy or porn films (usually the same thing).

But the benefits of masturbation are much the same as those achieved during sex. In fact, and I was charmed to read this in an article, though it seems an extrapolation too far, lower stress hormones mean you're less likely to stress eat, and therefore masturbation will help keep you thin. I'm not convinced by this, but I like the slightly convoluted logic. Are wankers less prone to weight gain? Answers on a postcard. Nobody has yet done a definitive study on the subject, though there's a surprising amount of speculation, and sex *does* burn calories, though only sixty-nine per session (such a marvellously fitting number).[10]

All for the pelvic floor

The pelvic floor is the group of muscles in your pelvis that stretches across from pubic bone to backbone and supports the bladder, bowel and uterus – all of which sit above it. Just like any other muscle group, the pelvic floor can sag with age, and if it's out of shape, this can lead to leaking urine, as well as pelvic organ prolapse (see box, page 249), where the bowel, uterus, bladder or top of the vagina start to bulge downwards and can even protrude from the vagina. Constantly going to the loo at night is also associated with lack of pelvic-floor tone and lack of oestrogen.

There is an expert for everything, and I went straight to Elaine Miller (also known as Gusset Grippers), a physiotherapist who specializes in pelvic-floor health and is also an award-winning comedian. The punchline here is clearly that you laugh at her jokes and try not to wet yourself. She says that the lack of accurate advice about our pelvic floors is an absolute scandal. 'The evidence we have is that most women should do exercises every day. Some women will have a non-relaxing pelvic floor (where muscles are too tense), and if this is the case then exercises might cause pain and not solve the problem. Then, you need to go to your GP, who can refer you to an NHS specialist physiotherapist.'

> The punchline here is clearly that you laugh at her jokes and try not to wet yourself.

You do not need to, nor should you, put up with incontinence. Address it right now or it *will* get worse. Too many of us see a little bit of leaking as our load to bear, and behave as though it's not a big problem. But then you may stop exercising and having sex. As we get older and more frail, it becomes even more of an issue. Elaine says that incontinence is the second-highest reason for women being admitted to care homes after dementia. After hearing this, I don't mind admitting that I clenched on and off for a full twenty-four hours!

The problem is that women are used to dealing with pads and mess. We are sanguine about bodily fluids. But, left to its own devices, a sagging pelvic floor isn't going to resolve its own issues. Nothing, as those of us with muffin tops are aware, will tone itself. We joke about not being able to go on trampolines after a certain age, but there's no reason why most of us can't, if we work towards good inner muscle strength.

As muscles, including the pelvic floor ones, become less strong around the menopause, there's no time to waste. I assume that you are doing those vital exercises right now – it's a reflex, like seeing somebody yawning.

A wealth of new, technically innovative companies is springing up, run by women, and pioneering products with a purely female focus. In the UK, Elvie are a market leader, having invented and brought to the market a 'hands-free' breast pump that sits in your bra, and, more pertinently for the older market, a rather brilliant pelvic-floor exerciser called simply the Elvie Trainer, which looks like a large, bulbous paper clip and comes with an app, rather like a Fitbit, but for your inside muscles.

Most women have a favourite place to do a pelvic-floor workout. For example, I spend a great deal of time on a train en route to London from Somerset and, although I don't pull out my Elvie App every time, I don't mind admitting it's an ideal moment for few internal press ups. Other friends find it's the perfect way for whiling away time spent in traffic. There are any number of apps which help you to remember and count them up on a daily basis, but I just do a few every time I remember – basically you clench and hold, as though stopping your flow of wee (but don't do it *while* weeing, as this can cause damage).

The Elvie might amuse, but you don't have to have a sophisticated app or a gadget. Elaine gives the best how-to I've ever heard: 'Pull in as though you're holding in a fart while breathing out,' she says. 'There's a scientific basis for this. 'A study looked at what command elicited the best pelvic-floor contraction. They ultrasounded tummies at the same time as giving different prompts to do the exercises,' she says. The one which had the most effective result on pelvic-floor clenching was that instruction. You can't say it out loud in a booklet, which is why social media has been so useful for spreading that particular message.' It is amazing. Try it right now, and feel all – *all* – the muscles pulling upwards.

There's a faint *Fifty Shades* vibe to the idea of those balls that you pop in and walk around while clenching, but Sam Evans says life is not like a porn movie. You won't have an orgasm in the baked beans aisle. Sorry.

Prolapse

Consultant Obstetrician and Gynaecologist CLIVE SPENCE-JONES is a member of The UK Clinical Guideline Group for the use of pessaries in vaginal prolapse.

We founded a group focused on prolapse management in 2019 to help educate the medical profession and women on correct treatment. It's one of those 'shameful' things which far too few women feel able to discuss, but there are superb and effective solutions.

Nobody knows quite how prevalent prolapses are, but up to forty per cent of all women may experience prolapse symptoms which affect their quality of life, and they are particularly common during the menopause years. Symptoms include poor bladder and bowel control, painful or uncomfortable intercourse, a sensation of dragging and lower self-esteem.

A prolapse is associated with embarrassment and fear; feel a lump in your vagina, and the first thought is that the bulge of a prolapse is cancer. Women also beat themselves up about not doing their pelvic-floor exercises. However, there is very rarely a serious issue.

There is good evidence that specialized pelvic-floor physio – ask for a GP referral – can reduce the sensation, awareness and aid bladder symptoms. It won't physically lift the prolapse back up, but muscle tone and quality of life will be better.

Topical oestrogen can help reduce symptoms of skin pain, and we also recommend using pessaries, which come in different shapes, such as rings.

They are inserted to give the organs support, are comfortable, and you can still have intercourse. Pessaries can either be self-managed and taken in and out yourself, or reviewed every six months. Surgery may be necessary, but only when other options have been fully explored.

Taking testosterone

Another – more pragmatic – element of the sex situation is the third hormone in the holy trinity of menopausal chaos. Testosterone, thought of as a male hormone, is vital for the functioning of the female; it's produced by the ovaries and adrenal glands and decreases throughout our lives. Testosterone is incredibly important for a number of bodily functions, including metabolism and thought, and it also increases the happy hormone dopamine and is therefore pretty useful for sexual arousal and orgasm.

'Most women don't realize that they need testosterone,' says our menopause expert Dr Tonye Wokoma. 'Even post menopause there is a tiny amount of circulating testosterone in the body. It's also good for tiredness and lack of energy.'

I did try it when I first started taking HRT, as recommended by my gynaecologist, but, aside from a faint blonde down erupting across my face, which I eventually had to have waxed off, I didn't notice much difference. Friends didn't just grow a beard, but have reported incredibly positive results, with libidos, energy levels and brain fog all improving. It's another example of the lottery that is currently most women's experience of menopause, with guesswork, good fortune and meeting the right doctor at the right time all part of the contributing factors for success.

Testosterone is even recommended in NICE Guidelines: 'Consider testosterone supplementation for menopausal women with low sexual desire if HRT alone is not effective,' they say. There is, says Tonye, also consensus from the British Menopause Society. Incidentally, they also say that there is trial data in women with Hyposexual Sexual Desire Disorder, HSDD, or testosterone deficiency, which indicates that testosterone used without oestrogen is equally effective and safe.

In spite of it being thought that a significant number of women would benefit from testosterone, there's not currently a licensed testosterone product for female use in the UK.[11] Staggering, isn't it? There are plenty of options for men, and that's what women are given, in spite of our completely different bodies and needs. It's prescribed 'off label' – which is to say, not the purpose for which it was made.

'Of course, it is closely monitored,' says Tonye. 'Clearly, we give different amounts to women, and it's important to measure and monitor bloods, as testosterone can have side effects, including acne, excess hair growth and even a deeper voice. There used to be a patch and an implant for women, which were considered safe, but withdrawn from the market.' So we are prescribed the gels or creams that are made for men, but in suitable doses. It appears that the pharmaceutical industry needs to catch up with medical advice and demand from women. (We are too weak from lack of testosterone to ask.)[12]

The psychology of menopausal sex

Women can't just switch on sexy. There's usually a certain amount of build-up necessary, and there's the question of how we're feeling. We've already talked about the general impact of negative body image in chapter eight, and feeling unattractive definitely won't help you feel sexy. If the world has one message on repeat for middle-aged women, it's that we are no longer top-of-the-range goods. We should retire without fuss to some quiet corner of the supermarket of life, where we can wait out the rest of our days, gathering dust, and without cluttering up shelves that might otherwise be crammed with fresher 'products'. If we aren't perceived as being sexy by society, it takes a great deal of inner strength to make ourselves feel so, especially if we're struggling with the physical side effects of menopause.

Professor Phyllis Kernoff Mansfield at Penn University published a study in 2004 entitled, 'Feeling frumpy: The relationships between body image and sexual response changes in mid life women'.[13] It was reported – and I think that this will come as no huge surprise, that women usually thought of themselves as being more attractive ten years previously. True fact. My forties now seem like a decade of supermodel-like beauty – relatively speaking. But, interestingly, how attractive you think yourself isn't dependent on whether you are menopausal. It applies at any time. Basically, the better looking you think yourself, whatever your age, the more you feel like sex.

As we all know, this is incredibly subjective. What I see in the mirror is by no means what my children see (the fun police and a washer woman) or my husband (a sex goddess?). But this isn't the point. Women's libido is based to some extent on whether we think we're good looking enough. A 2020 study looked at more than two hundred and fifty Norwegian women, and the less satisfied they were with their looks, the less orgasmic satisfaction they were likely to get from sex or masturbation.[14]

'Don't forget that your partner is unlikely to notice if you aren't perfect,' says Sam Evans. 'We're constantly told that we have to look a certain way. Once you realize this isn't true, you can change your attitude and gain confidence.'

> If the world has one message on repeat for middle-aged women, it's that we are no longer top-of-the-range goods. We should retire without fuss to some quiet corner of the supermarket of life, where we can wait out the rest of our days, gathering dust.

Knickers to it

I could have left you there, dangling by a slender rope of hope over a bottomless chasm of crap sex forever. But there is plenty of evidence suggesting that later-life sex can be fulfilling, and even better than it was in our twenties and thirties, especially as the swiftness to climax of younger men slows down and catches up with the slow-burn turn-on needed by women.

I included an example of this in the aforementioned anthology of erotica I edited, called *Desire*, where there is a brilliant story by Arlene Heyman. 'The Loves Of Her Life' features a couple of septuagenarians, clearly long married, preparing to have 'impromptu' sex ('Yes, dear, that would be very nice, making love'), an event that requires forty-five minutes of preparation, including timing the Viagra and the antacids, the use of K-Y Jelly and the in-head fantasies.

Such lack of spontaneity may seem unromantic, but deliberate investment in your relationship can bring welcome returns. Is there anything more cheerful than a post-coital male? Their joie de vivre (albeit short-lived) can seem almost undignified! Even we women, less directly hardwired from brain to genitalia, experience tangible emotional benefits from regular sex in terms of stress reduction, well-being and the physical workout for our oft overlooked pelvic floor.

But how to achieve that less-passionately prompted but imperative 'regular' in our long-term coupling, especially at a time when many women are feeling decidedly unsexy? On a country walk with the eminent therapist Julia Samuel in 2019, we were discussing the (many) challenges of long-term relationships, and she pointed out the importance of intimacy. As we all know, the longer you go without sex, the harder it is to have sex. So, she suggested, finding ways to regularly overcome the lazy brain of not bothering is to develop a good habit – like ensuring it's every Saturday morning. I'd take it a step further. Booking sex into the diary along with the weekly supermarket delivery seems a pragmatic approach, a useful way of ensuring it stays incorporated in your 'routine'. It's basic upkeep, like mowing the lawn or having your legs waxed.

There are many lame jokes about the lack of sex in middle age, and I suppose that Appointment Sex, as I think of it, may not sound as though you're hanging off the sex swing in bondage gear. But forward planning is never more important than when you're going through menopause. Some women are fortunate enough to experience a rush of enthusiasm for sexual activity when their hormones start to rollercoaster, but, for most of us, the impulse to have sex is on a sliding scale from 'less interested' and spiralling down to 'non-existent'. That said, it's a rare human who doesn't roll over after having had sex and think, 'That was nice, and really not too time consuming; we should do it more often!'

So, putting sex on your to-do list is proactive and constructive, and once you get started, it's fun. Having it set in stone also diminishes it as a late-night fret topic, because it's in the diary for Sunday morning (sober and without pressing responsibilities) or Friday (maybe a couple of glasses of wine to loosen up, and that end-of-week sense of liberation to spur you on). Maturity means a less-fanciful approach to what romance means, and the most romantic thing you can do in an enduring relationship is to value it enough to carve out some quality (naked) time with your partner.

A year after Julia and I had our chat, I read Caitlin Moran's bravely confessional book, *More Than A Woman*,[15] and was thrilled to discover that this diarized sexual encounter was actually a 'thing' – memorably termed by Moran as the Maintenance Shag, which is far more encompassing than my drearier Appointment Sex.

'I think every person in a long-term relationship knows the feeling when it's been so long since you've done it that the whole concept seems like some madly improbable dream you once had,' she says. Therefore, she and her husband book in lovemaking at a time and place convenient to them both. And, although I've promised my husband not to tell all or embarrass him, I'm prepared to admit that so do we!

Incidentally, although Caitlin and I are clearly of the collaborative persuasion, it doesn't have to be a recognized 'agreement'. I have a number of girlfriends who broadly agree with this concept, but it's more one-sided, and on the whole their husbands aren't necessarily aware that, 'It's Friday, so I'd better put out,' is what they're thinking as they pour a second glass of wine.

Sex may be less spontaneous, but it doesn't have to be less enjoyable. I think that making more of an effort is both pleasurable and respectful. In my twenties, I was a big fan of beautiful underwear, and it's a habit I got out of as I got busier, had kids and found myself in a decades-long marriage. When I hit fifty, suddenly I was once again toying with slivers of lace in the lingerie department. I eschewed the old, now greying, microfibre staples that had been my undergarments of choice, selected purely for comfort and practicality (not words you ever want associated with your sex life) in the intervening years.

It was out with the T-shirt bra and Uniqlo panties and hello Les Girls Les Boys, Noelle Wolf and my old favourite La Perla. Mrs Robinson became my mentor, and I came to the conclusion that great underwear is wasted on you when you're young and look good naked. Beautiful, feminine, sexy lingerie should surely be the preserve of the post-fifties, who prefer a bit of cover-up, but know how to work a bra and pants and hold-up stockings when the moment's right!

There are studies suggesting that sex in later life can be excellent, if you just put in a bit of thought. I read with great interest about an age-related phenomenon called 'sexual wisdom'. In a 2016 study looking at more than six thousand Americans, the authors noticed that, although sexual quality of life – they call it SQoL – does tend to decline with age, this can be mostly improved using what in my day was called 'a bit of effort'.[16] Or, as they put it: 'There was evidence to suggest that age may be associated with the acquisition of skills that can lessen age-related declines in SQoL (i.e., "sexual wisdom").' I'd say that this clearly translates to, 'Wear nice knickers.'

In terms of experimentation, I was staggered to come across a 2020 survey, which spoke to 2,381 (a strangely arbitrary number) over-sixties to understand their sexual habits as they grew older. Sixty-three per cent expressed an interest in BDSM and fifty-eight per cent in group sex. Really? Gosh. Sixty-nine per cent of men and seventy-three per cent of women said they think about sex once or twice a day – an average of seventy-one per cent, and – might I add – that's far more than me.[17]

Some women *do* have a surge of sexual desire around this age. 'A raging libido is very likely down to a surge in testosterone,' says Sam. 'But equally, if kids are older, you have sorted out your vaginal health, you've got the right lubes and you know what works for you, then there's no reason why libido and sex can't be better than ever.'

Who doesn't want to have sexual wisdom? I shall let my husband know that I am now a sex sage, and see where we go from there.

> Who doesn't want to have sexual wisdom? I shall let my husband know that I am now a sex sage, and see where we go from there.

Flipside

You can be as revved up as you like – moist vagina, adequate testosterone and skin-safe sex toys galore – and, if you want to, then enjoy yourself all by yourself. But don't forget the feelings of your partner, whatever their gender.

This is without question a time of life when men may have a lower libido as well. 'Men put on weight and tend to be less healthy around this time, drinking and eating too much and not exercising,' says Sam. They may also have prostate problems, and they have lower levels of testosterone after the age of forty.

There is much speculation as to the existence of a male menopause, and I investigated it while making my programme, even coming across some perplexing, though reasonably compelling data, suggesting that men can have hot flushes. I remain unconvinced about the whole concept, though accept that they have gently declining hormones, unlike women's more cliff-edge experience. Actual male menopause sounds like appropriation to me.

However, middle age is a stressful time of life for everyone, menopausal or not. Treat men (and women) with the same openness and sympathy as you'd like from them.

Finally, don't forget that you can still get pregnant. HRT isn't a contraceptive. And you can still catch STIs; you may run your own business and have paid off your mortgage, but genital warts have no respect for status and work ethic. I can't be bothered to point out the rising statistics of infection among silver shaggers (or whatever we're called). It's just patronizing. If you still have periods and – more to the point – don't know his sexual history, then use barrier contraception, ladies.

What women want

We've read a lot of clinical studies over the last few months, and, to ascertain what puts women in the mood for love, we conducted one of our own, by posting the question, 'What makes you feel sexy?' on co-author Alice's Facebook account.

This 'science' revealed that, for most women, 'feeling thin' was top of the list. 'Clean hair' was another erotic must-have, as was 'fresh bed linen'. But what about the men, you ask? These were mostly husbands, and were also required to be 'clean' and also 'soberish', although one puzzling answer requested that they 'have both lungs' and there were a couple of understandable requests for them to resemble Henry Cavill or Chris Hemsworth. Failing that, 'smelling of Tom Ford' or just 'freshly showered' was sufficient, and sexy behaviour included 'pushing a hoover round' and 'unloading the dishwasher'.

Top location was a hotel, but a downside of this option was 'the transactionality of it. Looking round a dining room and seeing all those middle-aged men on a promise.'

Claire

CLAIRE, FORTIES

Shall we take it as read that I find the person that I'm with attractive and funny? If that's a given . . . Being almost flat-stomached and generally fit, slightly tanned with clean hair, nice matching underwear, a bit pissed, clean sheets, tidy room (or a hotel room, which by default is clean-sheeted and tidy) – then add in an evening of flirting (even if you live with them) and lots of snogging. Also, I suppose you should probably add in knowing that he thinks I'm desirable and that my feeling sexy and up for it is reciprocated is important.

Alison

ALISON, FIFTIES

I think that, after thirty years of being categorized and pressured about sexual response etc., the menopause might actually be a time when we can be allowed to be interesting for other reasons and liberated from the whole matching-underwear shtick.

Frances

FRANCES, FIFTIES

I like it when he runs, bikes, chops wood and then, after cleaning up, smells good, puts on a clean white shirt and jeans, and kisses me. As I'm often a crabby old perimenopausal bag doing the recycling, and he often has a bad back or can't sleep, the timing is a bit like an eclipse, but when it happens . . .

The sex surge

AMERICAN AUTHOR OF 2019 BOOK *THE SEX SURGE*
JOANNA MERIWETHER, FORTY-FIVE

We joke about increased libido in your middle years, but it can quite genuinely take over your life. I started to notice what I believe is a surge in testosterone around the age of thirty-four, when I desperately wanted sex around the time of ovulation, but the desire gradually increased until it was all I could think about. This lasted until I was forty-two. Most of the women experiencing this are in their early to mid-forties, when the symptoms of the perimenopause are just starting to gently nudge your consciousness.

Thinking about sex the whole time is not pleasurable. I compare it to waking up in the morning and having the same radio station playing in your head for the entire day, and tuned to sex. I was frustrated, I couldn't focus on work, and it was hard to think about anything else. I'd walk down the street imagining how it would feel to have sex with almost every man I saw. On a horny scale of one to ten, I was eleven. I found that meditation helped a little, but, for the most part, I had a constant erotic earworm.

I searched medical literature for a reason, thinking that it was just an evolutionary thing: my body saying get out there and have one last baby. It appeared that I was probably suffering from a higher level of testosterone.

You'd think that it would be a husband's dream, but very few middle-aged men want to have sex all the time. Thankfully, my husband and I have a very communicative relationship. I told him what was going on and said I'd like an open marriage. He was kind enough to say that he believed in me and that I could make whatever choice suited me, but that he wouldn't be able to remain in an open marriage himself. Ultimately, he was more important to me than a month-long affair. Our relationship was very wobbly for a few months as we worked through our issues.

We compromised, whereby he was willing to have sex more frequently and I was willing to have less, but that was hard. There are still times when I feel apologetic and shamed about what I put him through. But we found our solutions. I also masturbated and read erotica and let all my sexual feelings come up while I did so. I started writing erotica, dressed in ways that made me feel sexy, wrote about sex as a holistic health issue, and I found foods, music and experiences that made me feel truly satisfied.

In retrospect, I realize that during these years I was grumpy, moody, perfectionist and telling people to do things my way. This is also part of what testosterone does to your brain: you're angrier and more single-minded. Some women experience a surge in testosterone and become more ambitious and creative or driven in other ways; I know one who retrained as a GP in her early forties, for example.

Now, I coach other women who have the sex surge – ranging in age from their thirties to their sixties. As soon as I started to write about this, I was contacted by hundreds of women who'd noticed suddenly increased libidos. It can be very disturbing and intense. Some have affairs, others may find themselves attracted to women, or bisexual women in long-term lesbian relationships have found themselves attracted to men again during this time. Some women even think they have a brain tumour, so alien are their feelings.

Ultimately, I am glad I had the experience. It opened me up in terms of my own desires. I'm more creative and honest with myself, and now I can talk about it and educate other women. I think heightened female libido is something which is thought of as shameful, lots say that their gynaecologists dismiss them. I think we're taught to feel ashamed, especially in mid-life when we ought to be frumpy and going off sex. But, if we listen to those ideas when we're going through the sex surge, it can really hurt our mental health. We need to find new ideas and stories and mentors for how to live with all kinds of libido levels at mid-life.

I also have a better appreciation of men and how they view the world. We lump them together and say they're all focused on sex, but when you are overwhelmed with testosterone, you have no choice but to have those thoughts. Of course, how we handle ourselves with those thoughts is the most important thing, for both men and women. Ultimately, I want women to feel comfortable admitting to all types of changes in libido and for women to feel socially accepted when talking about increased libido and sexual desire.

Rebecca Chance

AUTHOR REBECCA CHANCE, FIFTIES

Personally, I always assumed that older women had great sex. It wasn't even something I stopped to think about. I have been married forever, but I have always been incredibly flirty, and I think that one should flirt with everybody; it keeps those skills active, and one never knows when you might need them. I went to the London nightclub Koko a couple of years ago and stayed till the small hours. My friend Chloe was flirting madly with a very keen man at least fifteen years younger than her, and I started chatting to a young American guy in his late twenties and from Silicon Valley. We had a nice chat and a flirt and obviously nothing happened; I'm married, and I told him so. As I waited for my coat, he came up to me and said in a low voice, 'I just want to tell you that, if we had had sex tonight, I'd have fucked you through the wall of the hotel room.' People may wonder why I didn't slap his face, but it was so clear that he meant it as a compliment that actually I thought it rather charming. I said, 'Thank you, that's so sweet of you!' and meant it. Though, I must say, social mores have certainly changed since I was out there in the dating world.

CHAPTER ELEVEN

Hormonious Relationships

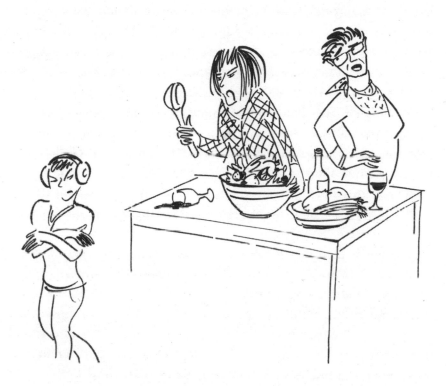

'During the years of menopause, elevated emotions, often negative or raging, might push us and those around us to the limits of endurance.'

I have a dream. Suddenly, I start to experience a hot flush. My entire body is burning up in the fiery pits of hell (feels like). My husband is watching sympathetically. 'Hot flush?' he asks, nicely, but not patronizingly, or annoyingly, thus balancing like a world-class trapeze artist on a gossamer-thin tightrope made from slender strands of optimism. 'Shall I open a window and fetch you a glass of water?' 'Thank you, darling,' I say. 'You understand me so well.' We smile lovingly at each other, and empty the dishwasher together.

Menopause isn't just about women. It affects everyone in your vicinity: partners, husbands, wives, children and friends. This last group is – I feel – more likely to constitute a pile of soft cushions for your emotions than target practice for sharp flashes of irritation. Originally, this chapter was going to be about partners, but then I realized that it's important to acknowledge and explore how all relationships might be impacted.

You don't need me to tell you that our moods impact on those around us. During the years of menopause, elevated emotions, often negative or raging, might push us and those around us to the limits of endurance. It should be no surprise that women are more likely to take extreme action in mid-life when it comes to relationships, whether in terms of divorce, abandoning long-term partnerships or embarking on same-sex relationships for the first time.

Clearly, there's going to be a certain amount of misunderstanding between men and women because it's very hard to envisage someone else's biology. But, speaking to lesbian couples, where both partners might be going through the menopause at the same time, the unique experience of every woman means that there are obstacles to their mutual understanding too.

If you have teenagers, who are by definition selfish and self-centred – this is science, by the way, not just weary observation – they may

> 'Hot flush?' he asks, nicely, but not patronizingly, or annoyingly, thus balancing like a world-class trapeze artist on a gossamer-thin tightrope made from slender strands of optimism.

be bemused, loathe you a little more, or possibly even be curious about your mood swings. Sadly, it's unlikely they'll recognize their own pubescent ups and downs and sympathize. They'll definitely only be interested if it impacts on them – whether it's taking advantage of your desperation for some peace, or responding to ill-humour by hiding in their bedrooms until you've left the building. In all of these scenarios, when it comes to our relationships with family and beyond, I think that menopause is ideally a time to breathe deeply before you utter a syllable, aim to educate, and look for those who might empathize.

We'll start with men, whether they are husbands, partners or boyfriends, because I am a heterosexual woman. It seems to me that not only are many men in near total ignorance of the menopause, but that this state of affairs can be damaging to our relationships.

Why on earth shouldn't men know what's happening to women's bodies? We are both human, after all. If they experienced the menopause, we'd definitely know about it! So, shouldn't they too be informed that one reason why their partner might be short-tempered, tired or finding them resistible is because their hormones are going up and down like pistons? This is emphatically not so they can attribute any displays of exasperation to menopause, as has historically happened with this and PMS. Nothing is more guaranteed to infuriate than being patronized.

Some men still have a very bad habit of using the vagaries of women's biology as excuses for their own behaviour. (Ref: 'She's bad tempered so I'm in the pub.') Nevertheless, might it be worth recognizing that part of the eye-rolling, sniggering and insensitivity on their part may disguise ignorance, concern and slight trepidation about what is really happening to their partner?

Since we women aren't exactly pouncing on the first signs of menopause as though it's the new Bond film, and our education is often as sparse as my knowledge of quantum physics, how on earth are men supposed to know what's happening?

I know that my husband is, on the whole, indifferent to the fluctuations of my hormones, unless they directly affect him. I have asked him how he found me during menopause, but unfortunately his answer was unprintable. For context, bear in mind that I believe I sailed through both my pregnancies joyously, one of the lucky minority for whom everything about gestation was a pleasure. Yet my husband describes me during those eighteen months as being unhinged, impossible to reason with and in the grip of dark and malevolent forces. Imagine then how he might outline a sleep-starved, terminally anxious, frequently bad-tempered and entirely absent-minded manifestation of me?

As I say, his response was unrepeatable.

Someone less generously-spirited might argue that men's 'mid-life crises', with far less biological excuse, have been tolerated and even sympathized with for all time. Imagine if they had a real physical reason to be distressed, and not just a burning desire to take up extreme sports, wear unseemly lycra outfits and enlarge their automobile horsepower to prove they've still 'got it'! I know there are reasons why men struggle, but it's a shame they take baring all so literally.

> Since we women aren't exactly pouncing on the first signs of menopause as though it's the new Bond film, and our education is often as sparse as my knowledge of quantum physics, how on earth are men supposed to know what's happening?

In a 2020 survey of fifteen hundred menopausal women and five hundred male partners, seventy-seven per cent of the men said that they'd noticed a change in their partner's moods, and fifty per cent that their partner had gone off intimacy. A further forty per cent noticed that their partner was always tired. Rather than being congratulated on their sensitivity and perceptiveness, these men often felt shut out. At the same time, a 2020 report by Avon, which they called the Global Conversation Deficit, found that twenty-six per cent of UK women feel either uncomfortable or very uncomfortable discussing menopause with their partners. I am surprised it's so few. I only asked my husband because of this book. It hadn't come up before then and I won't be asking again unless under duress![1]

Simply understanding what's happening can be a huge relief to us, so expanding that illumination to those in our immediate vicinity has to be the ideal option. 'The "not knowing" can often be one of the hardest parts for women,' says psychologist Dr Meg Arroll. 'I've worked with so many who've said that, once they have a diagnosis and treatment, their mood, and therefore their relationships, improve. Most partners are likely to feel left out and perhaps even a little worried that we're concealing something, and even rather hurt. But chances are, once everything's in the open, they are more likely than not to be helpful and understanding, or at least try to understand (or be red-flagged if not listening), if we do share.'

Clearly, not every relationship is conducive to chatting about hormones, and this can also be a personal or cultural consideration. NHS GP Dr Nighat Arif, for example, says that most men in the Pakistani community aren't informed about menopause. 'The fluctuation of hormones is a bit of biology which is poorly understood in Pakistani communities, as are the issues around it, so communication is very difficult for Pakistani women,' she explains.

'This is especially true in the perimenopause phase, whereby a woman might still be having periods, but the man will wonder (as do women) why they are getting menopausal symptoms,' she says.

'This impacts on sex life; sexual activity can be limited or non-existent, and having extramarital affairs is religiously seen as a mortal sin. I often find that men come to see me with associated problems, such as low mood, depression, high blood pressure, uncontrolled type 2 diabetes, and when I explore more, there are invariably stresses at home. They often describe the woman that they love as experiencing menopausal symptoms and are then very surprised, because only "old women" get menopausal symptoms.'

We asked men to speak to us about their feelings, allowing anonymity if they chose. Their responses were fascinating, but the overriding impression is one of misunderstanding. This simply confirms my suspicions, that the best thing we can do is talk about it to our loved ones as well.

Mark Smith*

MARK SMITH, FORTIES

I know very little about it and I think, for men, it's the last taboo. Anyone who lives with a woman is reasonably aware of periods and ovulation, and in fact I find them quite erotic. But when I think about menopause, I imagine my wife's ovaries drying up, she goes off sex, loses her libido, everything shrivels and she'll just want to knit for the rest of her life. Good sex will be out of the window. I think it's a bit 'ew'.

I don't think we realize that it's about the mind and the body; at most, I think we assume it's a bit of a hot flush by the fridge.

Also, and I don't think I'm being sexist here, but it's hard enough to know what to say if she's premenstrual. How do we address menopause? Do you wait to be told? Do you say, 'Oh, how awful,' or, 'I'm so sorry.' And then will she shout at us? We're living in ignorance partly because we want to! There's no good outcome.

*Name has been changed.

Simon Hartley*

LIFE COACH SIMON HARTLEY, FIFTIES

I remember watching Mum go through menopause when I was in my late teens. Dad had had a heart attack, but till then they'd had a very stereotypical relationship, where he worked and she looked after us four kids. There was a different energy to her, funnily enough, both positive and negative. She felt more masculine, in a way – it was an energy of doing and achievement and taking control. At the time, it made us feel very safe.

She always used to have cold hands and feet, and suddenly she had what she called 'boiling leg syndrome', which started in her fifties and continues to this day. She has her legs dangling out of bed as though they're on fire.

Talking to my female friends, there seem to be four aspects to menopause. There are the physical changes, like shape and hair. Then the emotional state, feeling low, and the mental state, unsure or a bit lost and with a lack of clarity but a sense of purpose. I've noticed a greater desire to contribute – as though the ripples of life get bigger, beyond the immediate family. There's also a spiritual aspect, thinking about mortality in a different way, with greater empathy, compassion and a sense of something bigger than us being available.

*Name has been changed.

James Whitaker

MARKETING DIRECTOR JAMES WHITAKER, FORTIES

I don't know much about what menopause actually is, but I believe it happens around the age of fifty. I know women stop having periods and they can't get pregnant, and I assume it affects the body, with things like headaches, sweats and flushes. I don't know what the moment of menopause is, but I do know the hormone in the female body – oestrogen. Would I know? I think, in my relationship with my wife, she'd tell me – I know when she's feeling off, but I wouldn't automatically put it down to menopause. If she's down or anything, I'd notice – she's naturally personable and positive. Her demeanour is very positive. I've never even heard of the perimenopause. I've no idea what that is.

Andrew Bowden-Smith

HOLIDAY-LET LANDLORD ANDREW BOWDEN-SMITH, FIFTIES

I don't have the exact terminology, but I know that there's a shift in the production and dominance of different hormones, which relate, in the main, to reproductive possibility. What do you mean, there is a moment of menopause? I thought it was an era rather than a moment.

Perimenopause is when you can get irregularity from what was previously regular. That could be having more periods than usual or closer together, or longer apart with no pattern for a while. Fuzziness in memory can be associated with it.

James Stephens

HEADHUNTER JAMES STEPHENS, FIFTIES

My wife is fifty, but I think she's a bit of a late starter with menopause. It's not really something we've discussed. I'm sure she'd talk to me about it, and I certainly wouldn't dare joke – I said 'PMT' once, and realized that wasn't the way to enjoy marital harmony.

Men should absolutely know about these things, but it's

probably one of those subjects which, because it doesn't physically concern us, doesn't necessarily consume us. I certainly didn't go through my forties wondering when it might happen to my wife.

Mid-life split

Although it's obviously not possible for everyone, having experienced parental break-up myself, I'm all for seeking balance in our existing relationships if we can. That said, 'diamond divorce' and 'silver splitters', where older couples separate, are both – I gather – a 'thing'.

Judging by the many letters I've received in my *Observer* agony-aunt inbox, women seem to feel a strong compulsion to embark on new challenges around menopause. Ending a long-term relationship rates quite highly among them. Interestingly, whatever age you are when you decide to call it a day, it's far more likely to be the woman behind the decision to divorce. Is it just me who finds that surprising? Popular mythology so often endorses the cliché of men finding younger models, but it's more likely to be females deciding that we're better off actually out of a marriage.

In 2017, an American analysis of over two thousand adults in a heterosexual marriage found that almost seventy per cent of divorces were instigated by women.[2]

'Wives report lower relationship quality than husbands, while men and women in non-marital relationships report more similar relationship quality,' said the lead author, Professor Michael Rosenfeld at Stanford University. Research also suggests that divorced women are happier afterwards, even though financially they are likely to be worse off.

UK numbers back this up. The Office of National Statistics (ONS) shows that the majority of divorces of opposite-sex couples in 2019 were petitioned by the wife (sixty-two per cent), the same proportion as the previous year. They point out that wives have consistently petitioned the majority of opposite-sex divorces in England and Wales since 1949.[3]

> I've no desire to throw myself on the mercies of the single silver-haired foxes of Somerset, or anywhere beyond my own back yard.

Professor Rosenfeld found that there tends not to be significant disparity between the sexes in non-marital relationships, and of course same-sex marriages have only been possible here since legislation took effect in 2014. The first same-sex divorces were recorded from 2015 onwards.

Now, clearly, I don't want to suggest that the menopause is responsible for the heterosexual divorce rate. Also, the ages don't quite bear that out as a hypothesis – although the average mean age of UK divorce in 2018 was 46.9 years for men and 44.5 years for women, which is perimenopause time.[4] But I'd certainly argue that it's likely to be behind or at least a factor in a fair few separations.

Much of the explanation for this is down to our maintaining traditional roles within marriage. 'Feminist literature on marriage argues that heterosexual marriage is not only gendered, but fundamentally asymmetric and inegalitarian as well,' said Professor Rosenfeld in the study. He quoted Jessie Bernard's famous words: '"There are two marriages, then, in every marital union, his and hers. And his . . . is better than hers." Even between the most enlightened of couples this is likely to be the case.'

I'd say this frequently still holds true. When I think about my husband, certainly a hard-working and much-loved family man, he is not, however, the one scooping up the socks and damp towels from the bathroom floor at the end of a hard day at the office. Yet we both work full time. I've no desire to throw myself on the mercies of the single silver-haired foxes of Somerset, or anywhere beyond my own back yard, but I'd be lying if I didn't admit to recognizing the appeal in choosing to be with someone who does have an interest in your dirty laundry – no pun intended.

Clearly, it might be better for all concerned that, if a marriage or relationship is utterly toxic and irreparable, it comes to a dignified end, and especially for the sake of children. But, with my agony-aunt hat on, I'd suggest doing everything possible to avoid this outcome. Divorce is usually expensive and extremely stressful.

My advice to mid-life women hoping for a better partner is that, relationship-wise, the grass is rarely greener. The act of divorce is hopefully, wherever it's playing out, a final act, taking place only when all other possibilities have been exhausted: couples' counselling, mediation and a final holiday together. And that last is no joke; I know a couple who lived together only in name for six years for the sake of their kids, and then, on a road trip to visit mutual friends in Italy, rediscovered their mojo. I find it utterly heartwarming when I see them in the local park, walking hand in hand, looking like teen-agers in love. So, never say never, especially if there's a vacation involved!

On the flipside, I know far too many intelligent women in London who got itchy feet, ditched their husbands and lost the house in Notting Hill and all their friends in one swoop, though, clearly, this isn't the average experience.

Despite self-help-styled encouragement to 'find yourself', you don't automatically skip off into a land populated entirely by hand-some and solvent fifty-year-olds without a trail of toxicity and three lorry loads of battered baggage behind them.

Plenty of women have found contentment and new partners after divorce, and good luck to them. But sexism in the post-menopausal years is never more evident than in the sphere of dating. A dear friend in her fifties, recently divorced, dipped her toe into the world of online dating. 'All the women were in their forties and incredibly glamorous. "Running a multinational company and looking for Mr Right" was the vibe,' she tells me. 'The men, on the other hand, were mostly balding, over sixty, and looked like the cat had got the cream. Positives tended to be along the lines of "own teeth".'

This is just a sample example, and I'm sure there are plenty of dating agencies with more balance, and swathes of exciting-looking eligible bachelors, but, even so, single girlfriends in their fifties tell me that it's not an even playing field out there, and at times it's a desert. And, unless your personal oasis is a man a good decade older, and who feels that he's lowered his expectations, then true love isn't necessarily a given.

As for the trend in dating far younger men . . . If it's for you, then go forth. I'm sure I wouldn't want to date a man half my age (and I'm fairly sure that this might be a mutual feeling), but I can't help admiring those who follow their hearts, or whatever other organ is doing the instructing. Of course, the most famous example is film star and author Joan Collins, who is by all accounts very happily married to Percy Gibson, a man thirty-two years her junior. On being asked about the age difference in 2002, she famously quipped, 'If he dies, he dies.'[5]

New relationships soon start to resemble old ones, and all too often the real emotional renovations required are internal rather than external.

Reinvention can be a path to personal happiness. Along with the huge challenges for couples navigating their middle years, there are equally large benefits for those who successfully do so. To those who separate and manage to companionably negotiate their way through their post-divorce years, I applaud you equally. Here's to a happy and companionable old age, whatever way you manage to achieve it!

Think of the children

As we lose the hormones that exist to help us reproduce, oxytocin, the hormone which helps us bond with our children also goes down.[6] Do we become less cuddly and more driven and ambitious? Perhaps more 'masculine' or focused in our outlook? We have spoken to women who say that obviously they still love their offspring, but in a more detached fashion, not that blind adoration you have for tiny babies or hapless toddlers.

'Once the hormones decrease, we may become less focused on

nurturing others, while more attentive to seeking fulfilment beyond family and relationships,' says Meg Arroll.

This is true. I have come across any number of post-menopausal women who are frustrated that their partners are happy to take the increasingly slow road to peaceful retirement, while they feel free at last, and want to travel the world. And, indeed, many husbands for whom the absence of a 'nurturing' partner comes as quite a shock! Just remember that children are incredibly sensitive to mood change.

'Kids, however old they are, will try to make meaning out of what's happening around them,' says Meg. 'The way in which they do this is often by blaming themselves; they do not yet understand the complexities of others' actions and reactions. They might moderate their behaviour subtly to try and stop Mum from being tetchy and angry. Over a long period of time without explanation this can result, for some, in a sense of anxiety.

'Look,' she says, 'women always feel a sense of guilt. We are not damaging our kids by being grumpy every now and again. In fact, that's humanity, and it's important that they understand people aren't always wholly formed of sweetness and light.'

I know that, in my late forties, pre-HRT, when my two were still very young, and therefore hopefully didn't notice as much, I was probably snappier than I might have been, because of lack of sleep, anxiety and stress.

I've already mentioned that my daughter thinks I threw a book at her during my perimenopausal years, and I stand by the fact that I think she's making this up. Joking aside, there is a platitude that a happy mother means happy children, which I take to mean that women should do as much as they can to be happy (and while enormously checking my own privilege and understanding that there are many things outside our control).

'If you do find yourself being angry or stressed, just tell them,' recommends Meg. 'Be honest, even if you think it's embarrassing to speak about the menopause. You don't have to mention your hormones. Simply acknowledging that you aren't feeling your best and emphasizing that it's not their fault is probably enough.'

The goal, as with husbands and partners, is to give an explanation so that those around you realize that it's not their fault. That said, when you're in the midst of a storm, you don't necessarily realize you are the one causing waves.

Talk to the teens

I asked parenting expert Tanith Carey, author of *What's My Teenager Thinking?*,[7] why it's so hard to talk to our teens about any discomforts.

66 Because we find menopause a difficult, intimate and sensitive topic, we often assume it's not a 'need-to-know' for teens. We tend to hope that our teen's biology syllabus will cover it, or menopause will come up in PSHE. Even if it does, it will still seem very one-dimensional to them. Kids need to understand it's an actual thing which is happening to you and other women your age.

The most common age to have a baby in the UK is in your early thirties, which means that many women are going through the upheavals of perimenopause at the same time as their children hit puberty. On top of that, research shows the task of setting limits for teens already falls more to mothers than fathers – and teens tend to be more antagonistic towards female parents.

So, all in all, the barrage of criticism, often mixed with contempt, which is part of the normal process of separation for teens from their parents, becomes harder to bear.

This can also make this period of parenting feel particularly tough. It is an age when we may already be feeling less confident and as though we're losing our bloom, while watching our daughters blossom – so we are often bearing the brunt of our children's adolescence at a very vulnerable time in our lives.

Obviously, the thought of their mother having periods sounds 'gross' to your teen, not to mention the fact that, at this age, empathy doesn't come naturally. Developmentally they have to be incredibly self-centred. It's a vital step towards cutting loose on their own and becoming independent. Teens also like to think they are the only people in the house going through anything difficult. So their first instinct, when they hear that you may be more tired or are having a tough time, is less likely to be, 'I can see she needs some rest,' and more likely to be, 'How is this going to affect me?'

Teens are still developing their 'theory of mind' – the ability to imagine what life feels like for other people – and the fact menopause feels a long way off to them means they are unlikely to be particularly curious about it or want to hear about it. Rather than be angry with them for being so selfish, you need to understand that it's par for the course.

Be matter of fact: rather than being dramatic about menopause, mention it as a fact of life. So, if your daughter is talking about her own period starting that month, mention perhaps that you haven't had one for a while and why. With boys, use some humour to say you need to remove some facial hair too, because you are also sprouting more of it as your hormones shift. Though your teen may not appreciate it at first, adopt a tone of 'we are all in this together', while reminding them who is the adult. Use it to empathize, open up conversations and ask questions. **99**

Friends are for life, not just for fun

Then there is friendship. Whether you choose to go it alone in later life and enjoy the benefits of independence, renewed confidence and new horizons, or work at reforming and reinvigorating your current relationship, there are those who will still be there for you through thick and thin. My girlfriends have been the life raft that's kept me afloat for nearly four decades now, and, while they were fun and frivolous and perfect playmates in my twenties, as the years progress, they have become so much more important than that.

'Women are hard-wired to tend-and-befriend,' says Meg. 'This is an evolutionary drive that has allowed us to stick together when times are tough and come out the other side. So it's no surprise that, often, lifelong female friendships are some of the most important bonds and sources of support that we have.'

I used to rent a country house with two lesbian friends, where I spent the majority of my singleton thirties, and where some of my happiest memories were made. At the time we would joke that we were going to club together to buy a house in Tuscany, to which we would retire in our dotage. It would be staffed by gloriously attractive nurses of both sexes, and we'd idle away our twilight years behaving outrageously, drinking martinis at breakfast and possibly nurturing addictions to the illegal drugs we'd avoided until then, or at least taking copious quantities of the ones we could get prescribed. Sharing our booty of antacids and sleeping pills, melatonin and antidepressants, and whatever else we could get our debauched paws on, could be one of our daily activities, along with cheating at cards.

Sadly, this hasn't come to pass, but I still think, as a dream, it's an excellent one. In reality, a close-knit community of people around you, who know you, accept your faults, celebrate your virtues and can prop you up when knockout blows come along, is key to a healthy, happy existence from mid-life and beyond.

So, as much as we expect our romantic partners and children to understand what's going on during menopause, it's also important to inform our friends. There is no better way of easing the pressure than airing and sharing your woes, and I've been amazed this last ten years to find so many women initially shy to confide, and then unstoppable when it comes to detailing the ups and downs, trials and tribulations of the hormonally unbalanced years.

> Sharing our booty of antacids and sleeping pills, melatonin and antidepressants, and whatever else we could get our debauched paws on, could be one of our daily activities, along with cheating at cards.

As seen in movies, from *Thelma and Louise* to *Beaches, Bridesmaids* and *Booksmart*, the pleasure women find in mature companionship is matched only by the intensity of teenage buddies who tell each other everything. I'd say it's even more satisfying when you're older, because you know how precious friendships are.

Alice and I toyed with the idea of calling this book *Help! I'm Hormonally Unbalanced*, but, for proof that friendships are imperative in this period, look no further than what you are reading: an enterprise dreamed up in a running group started among some middle-aged school mums and written by two of them. Our weekly outings, where we generally talk faster than we run, have been a rallying lifeline for each one of us at various times over the last five years: through divorce, mental illness, issues with children, death and health scares. If you do decide that, when it comes to your romantic relationship, it's out with the old, make sure that, when it comes to friendships, you treasure longevity.

I'm glad I was single

ARTIST ZOE GRACE, FIFTIES

I think I was fortunate not to have been in a relationship throughout my menopause. In fact, a girlfriend said to me that it was quite literally a pause from men.

Having always been about having a male partner – finding a boyfriend, having kids, then a family unit – I found myself grateful to be single, and for the women in my life.

In some ways I depended on my looks, as I had been a model in the 1990s. Then, suddenly and shockingly, in my late forties, people stopped looking at me. I became beige. Aged forty-nine was the hardest year, when I was coming to terms with how I was changing. Approaching my half-century I felt bloated, massive and unattractive, with my periods all over the place.

Because I was single, I could just cry. I didn't have to

share a bed with anyone, so I could throw off the sheets whenever I wanted to. If I woke up and needed the loo, I wasn't disturbing a partner's sleep, and if you're drying up a bit, well, it doesn't really matter. I was so emotional, and yet in a strange way I enjoyed my emotions and especially the anger. I found it all very liberating.

I almost split from my husband

NOVELIST FELICITY EVERETT, FIFTIES

As it happens, my husband and I are still together, and as happy as we've ever been after thirty-five years together. But, for me, the menopause was a werewolf-like transformation. Symptoms started when I was fifty. They came on gradually: anger, self-loathing, weight gain and depression.

It was very hard for Mark, but, as women know, there's nothing you can do about flashes of hormonal fury, although you feel remorse afterwards. We were going through a transitional phase whereby we'd downsized to an idyllic cottage in the Cotswolds, and my children were leaving home. In theory, we ought to have been blissful.

But I felt that, after years of nurturing, I was free to do more of what I wanted. I finally had the time to write, without interruptions from the children. Mark felt the same, but he wanted to do things with me. He'd been going hell for leather, working hard for decades, and, because I didn't earn as much, I'd done more childcare.

We fought over the most ridiculous things: what to watch on telly, how to arrange the house. Everything became a point of conflict. I did try HRT, but, just as I was prescribed it, there was yet another cancer scare and it put me right off. Mark thought that I ought to carry on taking it, which I took to mean that he didn't care if I got cancer! I felt as though something had snapped. I threw it away in a temper and drove away in a fury, screeching down our lovely country lane. We weren't the sort of couple who stormed off and then made nice again, so it was a big deal on the day.

That was the moment at which our relationship went right to the very brink, and also the turning point. Splitting up was the last thing I wanted – or needed, for that matter – and we talked very openly about our feelings. Almost a decade later, I am back to normal – better than normal, actually; more even tempered and less subject to mood swings. I mourned losing my fecundity and my femininity, and the only downside now is massive forgetfulness and stiffness. A generation ago, there wouldn't have been a resolution, and we'd have led a life with stilted conversation and resentment. I'm sure this way is healthier.

One partnership, two experiences

LGBT FOUNDATION MEMBER ANNIE CUNNINGHAM, FIFTIES

I think there is a perception of lesbian menopause that, because some of us share the same hormones, we'll understand exactly what a partner may be experiencing. I don't think this necessarily makes it a more harmonious time, because every menopause is unique.

I can't speak for all cis lesbian relationships, obviously, but, if you think about PMT within a same-sex relationship, you can see that your partner may be experiencing it, but you still want to take a long walk in the park to escape her when she is!

When my fifty-year-old partner Kate started to have symptoms of the menopause about six months ago – hot flushes and anxiety – we pretty much realized what it was right away. But we are an example of how very different experiences are. I was put on tamoxifen for a medical condition a few years ago, and went through menopause without any symptoms, so, actually, although I can see her poor face going bright pink, I don't know how it feels. I keep reminding Kate of that, at the same time as saying how very hot she looks!

A few of our friends have had huge anxiety; a highly paid professional became almost crippled with it, and went from earning vast amounts of money to not being able to decide how much milk to put in her tea.

Kate hasn't taken HRT because the symptoms have subsided for now. But I don't think there's anywhere near enough discussion about this side of menopause.

Once again, we rely on peer experience, which is very often out of date. There is so much false information floating around about HRT, most of which is based on outdated research. I feel that, as usual, we have to fight to get accurate information on medication that could make transformational change to many women's lives.

Nothing much changes, on that front!

I lost my laughter

GRAPHIC DESIGNER KATE CLARKE, FORTY-EIGHT

I don't know what chemical was involved, but, last summer, when I was forty-seven, and a year after I went through the menopause, I suddenly lost my sense of humour. Imagine how strange that feels. It was an entire personality change. I couldn't laugh. I kept putting on funny programmes to check – things which would normally have me rolling on the floor. Nothing. Did my family notice? Well, of course. I didn't find my kids amusing and had to keep explaining to friends. It was really distressing, and, as a normally jolly person, I felt completely different and quite depressed, lost, and like a smaller version of me.

I even went to the GP, and they suggested HRT, even

prescribing oestrogen gel, but I didn't want to take it. I ended up looking at nutrition and ways of boosting happiness via eating. I gave up caffeine and alcohol. I'm a little better, now I'm forty-eight, but I've realized that we all just come down to chemical reactions.

I assumed that it was negative

TRAINEE TEACHER ANNIE KENNEDY, TWENTY-TWO

My degree is in sociology from Newcastle University, and I decided to tackle the subject of menopause for my dissertation. The reason for choosing the subject is that I had no idea about it, except that, when I asked my mum, she said that it's something which is embarrassing to discuss because of hot flushes. In fact, I think she had quite an easy time – she went on HRT quite early on, and she says that it's her life saviour.

Before researching it, I couldn't understand why Mum and her friends would be awkward talking about it and get all embarrassed, when it was a natural transition. I personally didn't think it was something that should be dreaded, purely because I had no idea what happens, other than your period stops. But I was surprised by the lack of information, the toxicity of perceptions. We didn't learn anything at school about it – it never crossed our minds to ask. It was interesting, when I interviewed women, that they said going through it was the worst thing ever, and afterwards they accepted that it was brilliant and liberating.

CHAPTER TWELVE

Facing the Future: The Conversation Becomes a Chorus

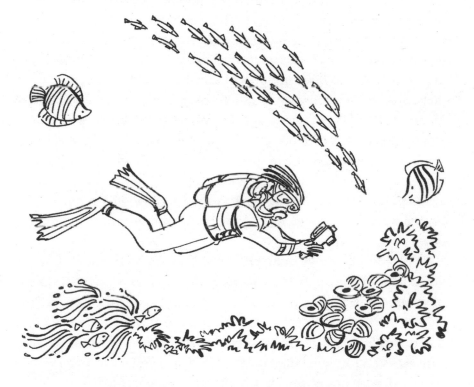

'We're finally celebrating this liberating time of life, when the world becomes our oyster, rather than our retirement home.'

We've failed in our mission if you're not feeling considerably better informed and less apprehensive about menopause, whatever age or stage you're at. Having put the myths in their place (mostly, the nineteenth century), sorted the HRT scaremongering and slotted the myriad of symptoms into some semblance of order, there's no reason not to step forth with a lighter heart and a better-stocked brain and bathroom cabinet. But being better equipped to survive the menopause is not enough. Who's up for a celebration?

In the award-winning show *Fleabag*, there is a blazing and heartwarming summary of menopause delivered by Kristin Scott Thomas. 'It may be the best three minutes of television ever; any woman over forty-five, or under forty-five, should have it on a loop,' said the *LA Times* in 2019. 'Menopause,' says Kristin, to an incredulous, martinisipping Phoebe Waller-Bridge, ' . . . is the most wonderful fucking thing in the world, and, yes, your entire pelvic floor crumbles and you get fucking hot, and no one cares, but then you're free, no longer a slave, no longer a machine with parts – you're just a person, in business . . . It is horrendous, but then it's magnificent . . . Something to look forward to.'

And she's absolutely right. For some (hopefully now ready to take advantage of the support available), the journey won't always be pleasant, but emerging the other side can be cause for euphoria. We said at the beginning that, throughout history, there have been too few women's voices on the subject of menopause. Far better to have kept quiet and suffered than been reviled, locked up or – even worse – 'healed' with one of the life-threatening 'cures' on offer.

When women do share their feelings about getting older, they often sound far less traumatized than 'experts' down the centuries have declared. Of course, there are acknowledged discomforts, and there are distraught case studies published by the doctors, but the official depiction of desperate, lust-ridden, shrivelled witches, burning with shame at being of no use to man nor beast has been hugely oversold. In reality, plenty of women have faced the concept of their advancing years with cheery equanimity and enjoyed a perfectly happy and productive later life. As our place in society improves, equality looms ever closer and we're 'allowed' to vote, have careers, and are generally in charge of our own destinies, it's often in the post-menopause years that we get to reap the benefits and come into our own.

> Of course there are acknowledged discomforts, and there are distraught case studies published by the doctors, but the official depiction of desperate, lust-ridden, shrivelled witches, burning with shame at being of no use to man nor beast has been hugely oversold.

Positive female voices about menopause start off as whispers, but, as the centuries pass, there is a gathering and public roar of acknowledgement that our post-ovulation years are far from a sad and redundant phase.

This has been pointed out by a few authors, who have taken the time to delve deep. It was acknowledged at various times that after the madness might come contented old age (and even a happy move towards being more like a man!), but women sometimes took it further. In *The Curse: A Cultural History of Menstruation*,[1] they reference American feminist and suffragette Eliza Farnham, who wrote about the menopause in the 1860s, calling it 'a time of "secret joy", of "super-exaltation"'. Hardly the 'mental asylum' mentality.

Then there's the famed women's rights campaigner Marie Stopes, who opened the UK's first static family-planning clinic in 1936. She argued that the 'crises' of a woman's life had been much debated by male medical writers, and perhaps the most artificially created crisis had been her 'change': the menopause. Of course, we had only just been given the vote when she dared put her head above the parapet.[2] I am reeling with surprise. So . . . the *men* were exaggerating?

Anthropologist Margaret Mead referred to our 'twenty-five years of post-menopausal zest' in the 1950s, and, in 1963, American psychologist Bernice Neugarten did a piece of research showing that many post-menopausal women felt better after the menopause than they had in years, feeling generally calmer and happier.[3]

In the last few years, there has been a cacophony of positivity. We're finally celebrating this liberating time of life, when the world becomes our oyster, rather than our retirement home. The menopause, having come in from the cold, is now the hottest of topics. We hear public figures, from heavyweight politicians to celebrities, speaking about the subject at every available opportunity. Yes, I'm not unaware of my inclusion in those ranks.

The always-admired Michelle Obama talked about her own hot flushes in a 2020 conversation with a friend and gynaecologist. 'What a woman's body is taking her through is important information. It's an important thing to take up space in a society, because half of us are going through this but we're living like it's not happening.' When Michelle speaks, everybody listens. If she can chat about her hot flushes as though it's no more of an issue than the weather, then millions of us are nodding along in relief.[4]

In 2017, the actor Gillian Anderson wrote a book with her friend Jennifer Nadal.[5] *We* is a manual for women seeking happiness. In it, she said, 'Perimenopause and menopause should be treated as the rites of passage that they are . . . If not celebrated, then at least accepted and acknowledged and honored.'

And Gwyneth Paltrow, who knows a bandwagon when she sees one, and always gives it a little added glamour, was positively pioneering in 2018 with her understatement: 'Menopause gets a really bad rap and needs a bit of rebranding.'[6]

The noisier the better, is what I say. We're following on from millennia of rigid-lipped reticence, or proudly proclaimed, but generally baseless, views from those who will never experience the menopause. For that reason, I find it puzzling when fellow females write weighty polemics suggesting that we need to stop 'going on' about it.

I'm happy to go on and on, and, in the process of making the 2018 BBC documentary and subsequently writing this book, I heard and read about hundreds, even thousands, of similar voices: celebrities, politicians, teachers, doctors, those sharing information on Facebook groups and websites, and those writing books. All of them were equally content to bang on about this too-long-buried secret. If you laid all the women now speaking about menopause end to end, I'd say we'd wrap around the world, and what a great advantage that would be. A planet encased by a crust of mature, wise and worldly women might be a better place for all of us.

Not only is it acceptable to talk openly and enthusiastically about the menopause, it seems advisable to point out the proven positives to later life.

Happier in every way

We are likely to be happier as we age. This is borne out by a great deal of scientific data, even though happiness is surely so subjective that it's near impossible to accurately define. Research suggests that our happiness throughout life follows – on the whole – a similar trajectory. We are cheery enough until we're sixteen, wibble around for a while, and then, according to a study using seven years of data from the Office of National Statistics, anxiety levels rise and happiness falls between the mid-twenties and mid-fifties, after which point it's upwards until about seventy. This is based on what's called 'subjective well-being data' – which is really whether or not you judge yourself to be content.[7]

Interestingly, although money is obviously vital, happiness is by no means dependent on being super wealthy, though I'd certainly love the opportunity to test out this theory with a few million pounds. I think the truth of this is best illustrated by a 2010 study conducted by Princeton University. They concluded that happiness increases up to the sum of US$75,000 (£55,000), but not beyond.[8] So, essentially, if you have enough to live off and enjoy a few luxuries, you're more likely to be happy.

This phenomenon is explained in a study conducted by psychologist and academic Katherine Campbell at the University of Melbourne. The study traced the happiness and health of a group of four hundred women, from their mid-forties to mid-fifties, for twenty years, and found that contentment grew along with the decades accrued.

'Women feel more in control of their lives and are still physically capable of enjoying their hobbies and travelling. They are often more financially stable and have less responsibility for children,' she said. 'They are free to enjoy the fruits of their hard work and are able to prioritize their own needs and wants.'[9]

Another Australian study, this one in 2018, with four hundred women aged between forty and sixty, also showed that post-menopausal women have a far more positive view of the transition than pre-menopausal. The authors pointed out that, 'Given the association between representations and bothersomeness of menopausal symptoms, clinicians should educate women about their expectations, and challenge their negative beliefs about the menopause.'[10]

Incidentally, there are also plenty of studies into confidence, and, again, the older woman very much comes out on top. Our confidence increases – and rightly so – with age and experience.

In 2019, *Harvard Business Review* reported a study whereby data had been collected from more than four thousand women and three thousand men since 2016. Only around thirty per cent of women aged twenty-five or younger said they felt confident, with around half of men saying the same. Remember that sheer insecurity of being twenty-five, an age for which I'd suggest the term 'imposter syndrome' could have been coined? We equalize by forty, but then, and this is the interesting bit, by the age of sixty, women tend to surpass men in confidence. Male confidence grows just eight-and-a-half percentile points between the ages of twenty-five and sixty-plus, but female confidence increases by twenty-nine percentile points. There really is a lot to look forward to and, as the latter proves, it's not just hearsay.[11]

Later life taking flight

Although reality shows and social media might suggest otherwise, it is entirely possible to enjoy a full and successful career later in our life cycle, and I don't just mean Judi Dench and Helen Mirren, who are always brought out and dusted off as older sex symbols and fine examples of how post-menopausal women can still work and, in Mirren's case, wear red bikinis.

A new and very relevant example is Kamala Harris, who became the first ever woman to take such elevated elected office when she became Vice President of the United States in 2021, aged fifty-six, and having previously been hugely successful throughout her career as a lawyer, district attorney and senator. Director Kathryn Bigelow actually hit the big time in 2008, aged fifty-seven, when she directed *The Hurt Locker*. Stylist Patricia Field was fifty-four when she met Sarah Jessica Parker and the pair were catapulted into award-winning fashion heaven during the heady *Sex and the City* years of the late Nineties. She's since been nominated for five Emmys. And Ariana Huffington founded the Huffington Post when she was in her fifties. Age isn't, and shouldn't be, an impediment to career goals and success.[12]

> I know from my own experience that, although my work goals may have changed, I'm far more industrious (and less hungover) than I ever was; I prioritize differently.

I know from my own experience that, although my work goals may have changed, I'm far more industrious (and less hungover) than I ever was; I prioritize differently. I still spend half of every week working in my beloved London, but I'm happy when I head 'home' to Somerset. I love what I do, but I also relish being with my family. There isn't the same sense of FOMO if I don't go to someone's party or the latest must-attend event. My contemporaries also seem to have a deeply committed work ethic, but also the ability to separate work and play quite firmly. If you can't put your foot down about family time when you're over fifty, then when can you? And it doesn't mean I'm any less ambitious, driven or focused.

Take note of money

Spend those pennies. Any money we have managed to accrue over the years – regardless of whether it's making us feel jolly inside – is vital to the economy. As lifespan and working life extends, the grey pound – terrible phrase – has never been more valued. According to a 2016 report from Saga Investment Services, the over-fifties hold 69.7 per cent of all household wealth in the UK. We are, therefore, the most powerful consumers – so it's high time we started flexing that muscle.

Not only are we spending on leisure services and travelling, but we're also the ones to watch when it comes to actively supporting employment and making money – and therefore holding up the economy. (It's at this point I fervently hope younger women will read the book and understand that getting older and a bit more wrinkly doesn't diminish your importance.)

A 2017 report by Hitachi Capital pointed out that the over-fifties are increasing their participation in the workforce – whether it be as employees or as self-employed. Approximately forty-five per cent of all the self-employed are over the age of fifty, they say, and business owners over the age of fifty provide employment to 9.8 million people. That hardly suggests that we're all sitting at home browsing stair-lift catalogues and counting the pennies we've hidden under our stained mattresses. What a shame that business hasn't yet woken up to the power of the post-menopausal pound![13]

We may be solvent and employed, but it will come as no surprise to discover that our power and wealth isn't being reflected in advertising or television. In fact, women continue to be represented as the same old drudges. A 2020 report from Enders Analysis (and founder Claire Enders herself is a glorious example of truly sexy maturity) noted the misrepresentation of women on telly, pointing out we are frequently and erroneously portrayed as stereotypes. For example, forty-one per cent of advertising showed women in a housewife role and twenty-eight per cent in an office role. But eighty-two per cent of women are the decision-makers when buying a new family car. That certainly isn't coming across!

It was also pointed out that brands which are 'gender balanced' or skewed towards women (£4.1 billion) are worth one billion pounds more than those tilted towards men (£3.1 billion). Now that's what I call headline news, so why isn't it writ large anywhere?

Changing face of beauty

Older women look fantastic when they're feeling buoyant and confident within themselves, but what joy to welcome the innovation of menopause beauty products. Even a few years ago, face creams specifically for menopausal skin were virtually unheard of. What's the point in making creams for has-beens? Happily, that's no longer the case.

The beauty industry, which does little product development purely from the goodness of its own heart, appears to be embracing the menopause as a new money-making bonanza. That's fine. There are positive overtones of change in the very fact that there's active investigation into the needs of menopausal skin, though some of the advertising leaves a lot to be desired. We don't all become born-again Victorian ladies in middle age, hankering after rose water and lavender bags! So much of the mature-woman packaging tends towards the floral – a little too redolent of nineteenth-century doctors calming us down with smelling salts and a good paternal talking to!

It's extremely heartening that menopausal skincare was flagged up on the UK *Vogue* website in 2020, and such hallowed reference certainly removes any lingering stigma! In that year, Alexia Inge, the co-founder of beauty website cultbeauty.co.uk, saw over three hundred per cent growth in the site's newly launched menopause section. 'When I started to research the subject, it really got me on my soap box,' she says. 'A lot of the products are rather lavender-and-lace in vibe, and some companies are definitely leaping on the bandwagon, but it's a fast-emerging category. The growing conversation shows that the historically dismissive attitude towards women's well-being is gradually changing; more are celebrated for their achievements rather than looks or the ability to give birth, and, unlike our grandmothers, we are retaining visibility and recognition later in life.'

When I browsed through the website, I found a reassuringly scientific, streamlined and emphatically stylish range available: VENeffect, DeoDoc (the excellent products for vulva and vagina which I referenced in chapter ten, see page 235) and Pause Well-Ageing.

Excitingly, there is even a movement against the term 'anti-ageing'. Some magazines are even recommending the use of the term 'pro-ageing' – which is about the acceptance that women would like to look the best they can, rather than twenty years younger. What with ageing being an irrefutable fact of life, how wonderful if this were the start of a sea change in the perception of beauty. I'm not quite able to be at the forefront of this particular battle. I suspect I may still be clutching the peroxide bottle on my deathbed, but relaxing the fight against wrinkles would be very empowering! In one hundred years' time, perhaps our crow's feet will be perceived as coveted marks of maturity, as they are with those handsome rugged older men used for advertising expensive watches, rather than a failure of lifestyle, genetics and personal maintenance when it comes to the female of the species.[14]

Shiny and bright

Intelligence can also increase with age. You don't have to think of post-menopausal years as being those where you constantly search your handbag for keys and your head for the right word. There is no reason to assume that your mind is fading, even if you were unfortunate enough to suffer from (or still do) the brain fog which can descend with diminishing oestrogen.

Neuroplasticity is basically the brain's ability to learn and adapt, and this continues throughout life. However, when we're older, we also have the benefit of what's called crystallized intelligence. This grows with age – it may peak around sixty or seventy – and is the ability to combine knowledge and experience to approach new problems, hence the wisdom recognized by the Grandmother Hypothesis (see page 31). This is also one of the many reasons why ageism, especially in the workplace, is so misplaced.

> **Intelligence can also increase with age. You don't have to think of post-menopausal years as being those where you constantly search your handbag for keys and your head for the right word.**

What a relief to learn that, after decades gorging on books for my BBC book show, activities like reading tangibly increase intelligence, keeping the brain active and slowing the decline of age. Not only does reading improve your mind and maintain agility, but it is linked to longevity. A study of more than three and a half thousand people found that reading a book for thirty minutes a day adds a couple of years to your lifespan. It's also said that reading every day means that you are less likely to develop Alzheimer's. Happily, I love reading and if it counts as brain training then all the better.

In summary, and with enormous satisfaction, I would like to confirm that the times are a changin'. We need to adapt too, and stop scuttling around in shame, trying to hide the evidence that we're no longer available for procreative purposes. Evolution has designated us far more valuable than the sum of our eggs, and it's high time we embraced that accolade and stopped being apologetic for reaching our perceived sell-by date. The first step must be to take control, steer ourselves comfortably through, and finally celebrate this rewarding phase in our lives that leads only to further liberation. I am over the moon that so many more women are standing up to be counted as loud, proud and menopausal, and thank goodness the conversation shows no sign of abating. I believe that menopause might just have been the best thing to happen to me. So let's redefine it as a fresh start and the gateway to an exciting future about which we are delighted to proclaim.

I love the confidence that comes with age

TV PRESENTER AND FORMER BBC ROYAL CORRESPONDENT
JENNIE BOND, SEVENTY

I had a relatively early menopause, at forty-nine, and it was a bit of a non-event, with a few hot flushes, and a sense of grief that I was no longer fertile. However, life in my fifties and sixties has been brilliant, for a number of reasons. I took quite a risk when I decided to give up my job at the BBC in 2003, when I was fifty-three, but suddenly a whole new world of opportunities came along, such as *I'm a Celebrity*, *Cash in the Attic* and a range of other shows. I'm still really busy, which means I'm lucky enough to be earning a good living, even at seventy. But I also have more leisure time – and the freedom to arrange my own work schedule. So, we go to Antigua for a couple of months each winter. I rather like the fact that I used to be dashing around as royal correspondent, trying to catch up with the Queen or Princess Diana, and now I'll be stuck in traffic or something but quite relaxed, because I know that the event probably won't start without me . . . and, even if it does, I have no boss to worry about!

I also take time to enjoy my beautiful South Devon home, overlooking the sea, and to hang out with my daughter and grandchildren.

I don't like the fact that I have gone quite wrinkly, which is one of those ghastly things that happens when you run low on oestrogen. I didn't take HRT because breast cancer runs in the family, and I'm rather envious of the friends who did, who have far better skin.

But, overall, I love the confidence which comes with age. I always now feel that my opinion is valid, I've got plenty of experience and the courage to say what I think. When I give public talks, I encourage people to go on challenging themselves, even scaring themselves, because it keeps your brain stimulated and your outlook on life young. I often tell people about an eighty-four-year-old lady I met who had just gone wing walking for the first time. She found it absolutely thrilling. So, never say you're too old to try something new and daring!

Changing the youth message

BEAUTY WRITER, AUTHOR AND FOUNDER OF
THETWEAKMENTSGUIDE.COM ALICE HART-DAVIS, FIFTIES

I welcome the advent of the menopausal beauty product. To be absolutely honest, few of them are effective, and none has as much effect on the skin as HRT, but I am glad that the skincare companies are recognizing this period of life. However, although the beauty industry talks about acknowledging the older customer, who they know is the one with the money and the inclination to spend on cosmetics, they are still massively messaging about youth. It's maddening to any mature or middle-aged woman that most of the advertising features ridiculously young women pretending it was a cream which helped them. We're not stupid!

That said, I'm not sure they're wrong to still acknowledge the youth message. Yes, we are seeing products supposedly celebrating age, and there is a kick-back about the term 'anti-ageing'; patients considering aesthetic procedures always say they want to look 'refreshed' and 'the best version of themselves', rather than just 'younger'. But the elephant in the room is that none of us wants to look older. That's the bottom line. Nobody wants skin sagging over their face like a deflated balloon, and that's why we're all using these creams and having treatments. Most of us don't feel on the inside how we look on the outside, and we try to counteract that.

There needs to be a shift towards accepting ageing. We all pay lip service to this concept, but I'm not sure how many of us genuinely embrace it!

I found new direction in my fifties

NOVELIST SANDRA HOWARD, BARONESS OF HYTHE, EIGHTIES

I had a bleak time in my fifties, feeling rather depressed and wanting to do something new; I was doing a bit of PR and this and that. That was thirty years ago, and it's not that easy for women of a certain age. As well as the low mood and realizing that the final downward slope of life was in sight, I also felt liberation from school runs and teenage problems. Then someone suggested I try to write a novel. The first one did very well, and I have just finished my seventh. Writing fiction is escapism, really getting into the characters and creating a sort of dream world, drawing on my own life experience to create the stories. Funnily enough, that downward slope tipped back up again. You realize that age is just a number, and what the hell.

This is the time to live our best lives

FASHION CREATIVE AND FOUNDER OF INSTAGRAM ACCOUNT @MENOPAUSEWHILSTBLACK KAREN ARTHUR, FIFTIES

I live my life for all the witches, for the women who said what they thought and got dunked in a pond for their trouble!

My menopause symptoms started aged fifty-two, with tingling legs. I started small gatherings to chat with my friends, where we talked about menopause – exchanging recommendations for vitamins and linen bedsheets! We tend to ask those in our circles, who look like us. Anxiety and depression meant that I had to leave the teaching career I loved, and I started to design clothing and teach sewing.

Then George Floyd was murdered in 2020 and BLM became globally visible. We'd already seen the murders of Breonna Taylor and Ahmaud Arbery, but that month of June was when the world really seemed to wake up to what black folk had known forever. I couldn't watch the video, but it was impossible to avoid the images.

One day that summer, I was sitting at my kitchen table with my sewing machine and I thought, Well, I'm black and menopausal, and my symptoms didn't take a hiatus just because of life events. I was upset, I felt for black women like me and I was moved to speak about the menopause, and how racial trauma can affect experience.

Racism is something that black women live with. It's ongoing stress: think about white supremacy, racial abuse and racial weathering. It affects well-being and, as an extrapolation, the symptoms of menopause – which could tie into why black women may suffer more from symptoms, symptoms that can start up to two years earlier than they do for white women.

The first thing I say if you are menopausal is, 'Google it.' It's quite shocking. All the images are of sad white women, and you can't unsee it. I have searched for research into our experience, and, apart from one 2007 UK study with twenty-two women, it's all about African-American and Hispanic women.

I decided to video my feelings about the subject, and I had the most incredible reaction from women, so I set up an Instagram account, @menopausewhilstblack.

Next, I launched a survey for black UK women, really for validation, and asked questions about where their parents are from and what symptoms they had. I thought that fifty responses would be a good chunk, but in the end it was well over two hundred. It's clear that black women were crying out to be heard, but we haven't been asked. It's not that our stories are necessarily any more or less unusual than women from other cultures, but nobody ever bothered before, and that's the big thing. We all have a unique experience; my hot flushes aren't as bad as some and I didn't have aching limbs. Some have tried HRT, whereas I explored holistic solutions. The GP offered me antidepressants, which I didn't rule out, but wanted to try other stuff first.

At the beginning, I didn't know what to do with the information, but then I realized, well then, I'd have to share it in some way, hence the podcast. I feel very strongly that this work is pulling me; I live in a way that shows women of all cultures, and especially those who look like me, that we can live our best lives through and beyond our menopausal years. My daughters – currently aged twenty-five and thirty, and who've witnessed and lived through every symptom I've had – need to realize that women who look like us can get to fifty-eight and be successful, desirable and relevant.

My menopause

WORLDWIDE BEST-SELLING AUTHOR MARIAN KEYES, FIFTIES

I never had it confirmed that the terrible depression I suffered for four years from about the age of forty-five was definitely linked to menopause. In retrospect it makes sense, because so many other women have talked about it, and I know that oestrogen is very calming; a dearth leads to anxiety.

I had two different doctors. The GP gave me HRT and my psychiatrist, who was a young man, the antidepressants, but he never suggested that it might be hormonal, and the GP didn't make the connection that I could be feeling this crazy because of the start of menopause.

It just kind of highlights how unimportant the issue of menopause is, because it affects women of a certain age, and nobody cares. We aren't just invisible, but almost scorned. There's something very unattractive about the idea of a menopausal woman. And the whole thing is that we are either mocked or we are shunted away. There isn't really a place for us in a world where everyone's supposed to be lovely and young and fertile and productive.

LOOKS: LOSING MY INVISIBILITY

I never felt that I fitted the template of a sexy or an attractive woman. I've always been the person who is ignored in the queue in the shop. I'm short and I have a meek face. Shopkeepers look at me and they think, 'She'll be no trouble. I'm going to deal with the trickier people first.'

So, in some ways, and this is going to sound weird, but I feel more attractive now than I did in my twenties. I suppose I was probably much more objectively attractive then, but I hated myself so much and I self-sabotaged all the time, so it was no good with me. Now, I'm fifty-seven, and I know I scrub up well. I can be far kinder about my looks now.

Partly it's because I'm more confident, better able to stand up for myself and carve out my place in a conversation. In myself I feel happier. I don't think of myself just as looks. I know that I tend to be kind. I'll go out of my way to make people feel comfortable, that my looks are part of a package of a decent person.

And, I don't know what you can make of this, but I take a huge amount of care of my appearance now. I have Botox, I have fillers, I care about my skin and I have extensions in my hair. It matters to me. I think because of that I don't feel less visible now, which is nice.

When you're younger, you have this idea that looks are everything. However stunning you are, when you're older, people aren't drawn to you by beauty alone. We want more. If you're not kind or entertaining or clever, or if you aren't present, it doesn't matter how physically beautiful you are. It's like all the things our mothers told us are true – to be beautiful on the inside is important too.

THE HRT CHOICE

It's interesting that women aren't always given a choice in this situation, that a GP or gynaecologist might say, 'Right, that's it. You've had enough. Now I won't give you any more,' after five or six years. I think that's an infantilizing attitude to the woman. Surely we have some say in it? This all comes back to the idea of a menopausal woman not being a full human being, someone who doesn't have full agency, and that really needs to be looked at.

I was talking to my sister about this last night. I know there are lots of scares about HRT. But, for me, the thought of returning to that state of mind I was in . . . I can't describe how frightening it is.

AFTER THE MENOPAUSE

I know what I want and I love my job, and it's all I want to do in terms of a career. I will make time for people, and meeting up with those whom it's lovely to be around, and that's a gift to myself that I wouldn't have given twelve years ago when it was all about the work and proving that I'm productive and worthwhile.

I was always so hard on myself, feeling guilty about any time I took off. It was insane when I think about it. We're all told we're nothing without our jobs and our drive and our five-year plan, and it's so lovely not to put that pressure on myself any more. I am less driven. That itself is a power.

A lot of caring about what other people think falls away, but it doesn't go entirely, and I think it's important to state that. There are no absolutes about being a human being. Every feeling I've ever had is still available to me.

In general, I'm far better at being more bold, more daring, and another thing is I feel as though I've fallen in love with people again, and with women in particular. I find there are so many sound women who make me laugh and are just hilarious. They don't sugar-coat things. I feel there's a huge – in me – ability to love, which maybe wasn't available before. I want new friends, and to meet people and think, God, you're lovely, let's stay in touch. I worked so hard in my thirties and forties that maybe I didn't have the time in the same way.

IF MEN HAD THE MENOPAUSE

Well, between the years of forty-five and fifty-five, they'd have ten years off work on full pay. When they were finally through, there'd be a massive party about their transition through to the Great Wise Stage of their lives. (If they had periods, there would be a Period Institute, they'd have three days off work every month and a chocolate and painkiller allowance.)

Whereas menopausal women are regarded as creatures to be mocked. People are always saying, 'Haha, she broke loads of plates and now she's refusing to do the ironing for us. She's going through The Change. It's hilarious.' It's no way to treat people who are going through something enormous and debilitating.

THE CONVERSATION

It needs to be talked about until it becomes the norm, and not something shameful or risible. It's just something which needs to be part of the mainstream. There's no need for it to be secret.

Motivation

PRESENTER AND FOUNDER OF THE MID·POINT PODCAST
GABBY LOGAN, LATE FORTIES

What motivated me to do my podcast is the thought that, when you get to your late forties, you still have goals and aspirations, but think that it's too late. Your confidence is gone. But we're going to be working till our mid-seventies, so we may as well do things we enjoy and things which fulfil us. We shouldn't be afraid; we have wisdom and experience to share. Yes, when you're around youth and youth culture, it's tempting to feel that you're old hat. In fact, a friend called me on my forty-seventh birthday and said I'd reached the age at which your mindset is fixed. Either you've achieved everything, or you never will. I said I'm not sure I'm going to agree with that. I wanted listeners to feel positive.

MENOPAUSE

I've started reading a bit more about menopause, and your ears prick up when you hear things – like when you're trying to get pregnant you notice information about the subject everywhere. You don't want a self-fulfilling prophecy when it comes to symptoms, but it's good to understand this kind of thing. I want to be aware: are my supplements right, am I doing the right exercise? Thankfully, these conversations are far more open now.

Over the last year, I've noticed my periods are less regular – it's one every couple of months, and, for all my fertility issues, my periods have always been regular. That's the only tangible thing I've seen.

Sometimes I look at my skin and wonder whether it's drier and if there's more downy hair, and my hair wasn't as thick last year, but then it came back again.

LOOKS

I remember someone saying to me, when I was in my twenties and she was in her forties, that she felt relief that she could walk down the street and not be wolf-whistled at. I know what she meant now. Looks are no longer defining.

In addition, you start to see the beauty in age, the women who age and feel content and confident, and I think the quirkier the better. Of course there's something about a teenager with flawless skin, which is so fresh and lovely, but character comes with age; we all wore too much make-up when we were teenagers.

If people want to change things and have surgery to feel better, then that's the world we live in, but I think there's something reassuring about feeling that you've accepted your face. Look to other role models – those you know are in their late fifties, and who look great but have lines and wrinkles.

MEMORY

As a live broadcaster, if I'm struggling to grapple with a name, I wonder whether that's a sign of menopause, and am more mindful – writing things down and having notes, just in case. But, as you get older, your brain is so full anyway, especially with teenage children. It seems unfair that this happens when you have challenging young adults in the house. At this time of life, multi-tasking is off the scale, and your relationship with kids changes. It's lovely and vibrant, but far more challenging. It's like being a barrister, having to create an argument which satisfies them.

Epilogue

Having been through menopause and emerged to find the sun still shining on the other side, I can assure you that it is not the inescapable black hole I originally assumed. Instead, equipped with knowledge and the right tools, menopause can be an ultimately enriching passage, culminating in a more confident and happier life, despite the unavoidable aches and pains and irritating symptoms of ageing.

I think I'm probably healthier, happier and fitter than I've ever been, barring three months in my thirties when I fancied a man at the local gym and barely left the running machine for fear of missing him.

Along with celebration, we need to start demanding change in the treatment, or should that be mistreatment, of so many women after centuries of misinformation and malpractice. I never want to hear another anecdote about a doctor's appointment that ends with the GP saying he or she doesn't agree with HRT, or fobbing the patient off with a prescription for antidepressants.

> I think I'm probably healthier, happier and fitter than I've ever been, barring three months in my thirties when I fancied a man at the local gym and barely left the running machine for fear of missing him.

If this book highlights anything, it should be the importance of a Best Practice GP Guide to Menopause, new guidelines for employers and the same amount of time devoted to the topic on the school syllabus as there is to puberty. This trio of knowledge might help bring an end to the sense of terror, embarrassment and ignorance many of us feel at the onset of what's simply a mid-life readjustment.

A modern interpretation of traditional Chinese medicine is that our post-menopausal years might be viewed as a Second Spring, which Chinese medicine practitioner Katie Brindle tells me is a metaphor used extensively to describe this time. I won't labour the point, as the imagery is pretty obvious: green shoots, fresh approaches, renewed vigour and so on.

I even found a passage describing the process, which she says appears to derive from a translation of the Yellow Emperor's Classic of Internal Medicine (2600 BC).

At seven times seven a woman's heavenly dew wanes;
the pulse of her Conception channel decreases.
The Qi that dwelt in the baby's palace moves upward into her
    heart,
and her wisdom is deepened.

It is a shame, of course, to lose one's heavenly dew, but the idea of becoming more powerful, knowledgeable and with stacks of deep wisdom is one that I, and hopefully all of you, eagerly anticipate.

Understanding the historical culture that's led us down our current cul-de-sac of fear and ignorance is half the fight. Celebrating future freedom requires a further shift away from the status quo. Navigating your way across this occasionally choppy sea will be infinitely easier if you are fuelled by vigour and excitement about this entirely natural and, dare I say, welcome period of no periods.

I certainly do not mourn the monthly pains, the inconvenience of buying expensive and ecologically unfriendly sanitary products (though there are emerging alternatives) and being in charge of contraception (I occasionally read about the male pill, but, really, why would they?). Instead, I'm singing a heavenly (though dew-less) hallelujah for my reprieve from biology. It means that I can concentrate on other priorities.

We need to ensure that society celebrates and accepts women at every stage of their lives. To have a span of years which might exceed our reproductive decades is precious time into which we can pack our ambitions and fulfil our outstanding dreams.

Returning to the Grandmother Hypothesis, the more I think about it, the more I believe that modern society is possible only because of the gift of menopause.

Rather than wishing we could remain potential baby-makers for longer, we need to re-evaluate our position. Granted, fertility is a relatively short stage of our lives. But it's made difficult by society, not by our limited biology. There is much written about women being selfish and postponing children for the sake of their career. But this is because everything is constructed around men. Education, career, marriage, babies . . . promotion and retirement: it's all very linear, because men aren't curtailed by biology and can procreate at any time.

So why aren't we demanding that women can choose to have babies at the best time for our health or circumstances and be supported in that endeavour? Instead of flexible childcare and support in our most fertile years, we're offered options like egg-freezing programmes in work contracts to encourage us to remain in the office. Do we really need to medicalize baby-making, take strong drugs and put our eggs into cold storage just so that we can also get good jobs and not be overlooked for promotion?

Restoring failing ovaries is a future possibility. Consultant paediatric oncologist Sheila Lane at Oxford University Hospitals NHS Foundation Trust is a child cancer specialist leading a treatment programme for children and young adults that can reverse the early menopause sometimes caused by chemotherapy. Here, they freeze ovarian tissue, which can then be re-implanted to restore function and fertility. It is staggeringly clever. In theory, this technology might one day be used to replace HRT and keep our natural oestrogen levels flowing for longer. But do we really need this 'solution' if it's purely to extend fertility? If we're in the lucky majority whose menopause arrives naturally in mid-life, it's surely better to pass through the stage with the proper support? It's a reality to embrace, not flinch from.

It's wonderful that women can already – should they wish to – have babies in their fifties and beyond, and great if it's a conscious choice. But, and I'm sure that others must have pointed this out, society itself needs to adapt to the fact that we have a healthy window in which to procreate; it needs to support us through that and then encourage us as we move on and flourish.

This is a far better way for women's lives to evolve, harnessing the value we have to offer as mature, confident and far wiser adults. So why not make it possible for us to do so by ending the negative imagery and investing in better education, support and opportunities for girls and women as they move through their biological lives? This really is a final frontier when it comes to women reaching their full potential. Educate everybody, offer the right support and watch society and the economy flourish, in the company of far happier and more fulfilled women.

Yes, the menopause is The Change, but one for the better. Watch out for the menopausal woman, for she is driven and passionate, and she seeks pastures new. Or, as the inimitable Caitlin Moran said in 2020 (and to paraphrase), 'Men's midlife crises involve a motorbike, a tattoo or remarrying. Women get PhDs.'[1]

I know that I am bolder, more enterprising and certainly less insecure than I have ever been. And the evidence points to many women in their fifties becoming equally fearless, ditching bad relationships, embarking on new careers and reinventing themselves both socially and biologically by adopting healthier lifestyles and emotional resilience for the second phase of their lives.

> Watch out for the menopausal woman, for she is driven and passionate, and she seeks pastures new.

Renewed confidence is the greatest gift, allowing you to find peace in your own company; to wear what you like rather than let the vagaries of fashion dictate wardrobe choices; to enjoy more intimate and honest relationships with your friends and family; and to find laughter and wisdom where others see only the tragedy of leaving youth behind. I know nowadays how to wring every last ounce of pleasure from each breathing moment and intend to keep doing so, as healthily and heartily as possible, for as many more decades as my beating heart allows.

As my gender stands taller (though not yet tall enough) in the sunlight, with women's issues on the menu as never before, it's high time we heaved this last instalment of our biological cycle into the daylight where it belongs. Negative assumptions about menopause represent the last great barrier to full equality.

I've never sympathized with King Canute's foolishness, and, by accepting that we can't turn back tides or time, we can focus instead on leading healthier, more illuminated lifestyles, and so make the most of these promising decades that lie ahead.

Confronting your worst fears can only make you stronger, and that's how my own chapter closes. The aim is an ambitious one, to rebrand the menopause as a fresh start and a new phase of life, a Second Spring, with all the bursting shoots of inspiration and exciting activity that that vision conjures up, rather than seeing your periods stopping as the first nail in a rapidly slamming coffin lid. Thousands of years of counterarguments need to be totally dismissed as we rise like the proverbial phoenix from the ashes of our youth and fertility. We can't afford to waste another second.

Notes

Preface

1. https://www.elle.com/culture/movies-tv/news/a27960/amy-schumer-tina-fey-last-fuckable-day/
2. https://www.telegraph.co.uk/comment/4255243/Not-an-empty-husk.html
3. https://www.poetryfoundation.org/poems/50428/song-fear-no-more-the-heat-o-the-sun-
4. https://www.britannica.com/story/just-how-old-is-homo-sapiens
5. https://marine-conservation.org/media/shining_sea/place_wpacific_mariana.htm

Introduction

1. https://www.prnewswire.co.uk/news-releases/menopausal-women-being-prescribed-inappropriate-antidepressants-survey-824831396.html

Chapter One

1. Reuben, David. *Everything You Always Wanted to Know About Sex* (*But Were Afraid to Ask)*, David McKay Company, Inc., New York, NY, 1969, updated 1999
2. Leunissen, Mariska. *From Natural Character to Moral Virtue in Aristotle*, Oxford University Press, New York, NY, 2017
   Muscat Baron, Yves. *History of the Menopause*, University of Malta, Msida, 2013
3. Dean-Jones, L. 'Menstrual Bleeding According to the Hippocratics and Aristotle' in *Transactions of the American Philological Association*, vol. 119, 1989, pp. 177–91.

4. Amundsen, Darrel W. & Diers, Carol Jean. 'The Age of Menopause in Medieval Europe' in *Human Biology*, vol. 45/4, 1973, pp. 605–12.

5. http://scihi.org/trotula-of-salerno-and-womens-health-in-the-middle-ages/
https://departments.kings.edu/womens_history/trotula.html#:

6. Amundsen & Diers, 'The Age of Menopause'
https://www.huffpost.com/entry/8-reasons-why-hildegard-matters-now_b_2006626?guccounter=1&guce_referrer=aHR0cHM6Ly93d3cuZ29vZ2xlLmNvbS8&guce_referrer_sig=AQAAAMHMZ55K0RNL-hMxER3u0jjqQ8pjcSwwtFefiCufqcde7PCPSYNPbTvl-pPYXbCaFPY9RExId9Nb7GjHmB9tYj8Ejci8dVLbb8_W6cfwRwld-GVT468ilF50iaY3GvYnXz_L-bE8Xfy9i9PAzyApH3jrSveXQeGw8mCk6KyjoigY
https://www.spiritualtravels.info/spiritual-sites-around-the-world/europe/the-hildegard-of-bingen-trail-in-germany/the-life-of-hildegard-of-bingen/

7. Godfrey, Jessica E. *Attitudes Toward Post-Menopausal Women in the High and Late Middle Ages, 1100–1400*, Xlibris Corporation, Bloomington, IN, 2011

8. https://micro.magnet.fsu.edu/optics/timeline/people/magnus.html

9. Stolberg, Michael. 'A Woman's Hell? Medical Perceptions of Menopause in Preindustrial Europe' in *Bulletin of the History of Medicine*, vol. 73/3, 1999, pp. 404–28.
This publication offered staggering insights into how women were perceived at this time.

10. Minkowski, W.L., 'Women healers of the middle ages: selected aspects of their history', *Am J Public Health*, 1992, vol. 82/2, pp. 288–95

11. Foxcroft, L. *Hot Flushes, Cold Science: A History of the Modern Menopause*, Granta, London, 2011, p. 66

12. https://www.bl.uk/collection-items/the-discovery-of-witchcraft-by-reginald-scot-1584
https://www.historic-uk.com/CultureUK/Witches-in-Britain/

13. Stolberg, 'A Woman's Hell?'

14. https://blogs.scientificamerican.com/science-sushi/evolution-out-of-the-sea/
https://www.smithsonianmag.com/science-nature/becoming-human-the-evolution-of-walking-upright-13837658/

15. Moore, Alison. 'The French Elaboration of Ideas about Menopause, Sexuality and Ageing' in *French History and Civilization*, vol. 8, 2019, pp. 34–50

16. https://www.etymonline.com/word/menopause

17. Van Keep, P., Notelovitz, M. (eds.). *The Climacteric in Perspective: Proceedings of the Fourth International Congress on the Menopause, held at Lake Buena Vista, Florida, October 28–November 2, 1984,* MTP Press, Lancaster, 1986
Foxcroft, *Hot Flushes*, p. 68
Stolberg, M. '"Stufenjahren" zur "Menopause". Das Klimakterium im Wandel der Zeit, ['From "anni climacterici" to "menopause". The historical roots of the concept of "climacteric"'] in *Wurzbg Medizinhist Mitt.*, vol. 24, 2005, pp. 41–50

18. Smith-Rosenberg, Carol. 'Puberty to Menopause: The Cycle of Femininity in Nineteenth-Century America' in *Feminist Studies*, vol. 1(3/4), 1973, pp. 58–72

19. Smith, W. Tyler. 'The Climacteric Disease in Women; A Paroxysmal Affection Occurring at the Decline of the Catamenia' in *London Journal of Medicine*, vol. 1, no. 7, 1849, pp. 601–9

20. Smith-Rosenberg, 'Puberty to Menopause'
Wiley, Margaret. *Women, Wellness, and the Media,* Cambridge Scholars, Newcastle upon Tyne, 2008

21. Tilt, E. J. *The Change of Life in Health and Disease: A Practical Treatise on the Nervous and Other Affections Incidental to Women at the Decline of Life,* J. Churchill, London, 1857, p. 37

22. Wiley, *Women, Wellness, and the Media,* p. 233

23. Showalter, Elaine, *The Female Malady: Women, Madness, and English Culture, 1830–1980,* Penguin, London, 1987

24. Smith-Rosenberg, 'Puberty to Menopause'

25. Smith, 'The Climacteric Disease in Women'

26. Tilt, E. J. *A Handbook of Uterine Therapeutics and of Diseases of Women,* J. Churchill, London, 1868
Tilt, *The Change of Life*

27. Lupton, M. J., Toth, E., Delaney, J. *The Curse: A Cultural History of Menstruation,* University of Illinois Press, Champaign, IL, 1988, p. 217
https://www.balancehormoneoklahoma.com/blog/the-history-of-menopause

28. McCrea, F. 'The Politics of Menopause: The "Discovery" of a Deficiency Disease' in *Social Problems*, vol. 31/1, 1983, pp. 111–23

29. https://www.livescience.com/54682-is-penis-envy-real.html

30. https://www.theatlantic.com/magazine/archive/2019/10/the-secret-power-of-menopause/596662/
    Lupton, et al, *The Curse*, p. 220

31. Callahan, Joan C. (ed). *Menopause: A Midlife Passage*, Indiana University Press, Bloomington, IN, 1993, p. 51

32. Bookspan, Phyllis T. and Kline, Maxine. 'On Mirror and Gavels: A Chronicle of How Menopause Was Used as a Legal Defense Against Women' in *Indiana Law Review*, vol. 32/4, 1999, pp. 104–10
    https://journals.iupui.edu/index.php/inlawrev/article/view/3382
    https://mckinneylaw.iu.edu/ilr/pdf/vol32p1267.pdf

33. de Beauvoir, Simone (Author); Borde, Constance (Translator). *The Second Sex*, Vintage Classics, London, 2010 edition, Kindle Location 12669; 12708
    de Beauvoir, Simone. *The Coming of Age*, W. W. Norton & Company, London, 1996 edition

34. Wilson, Robert. A. *Feminine Forever*, M. Evans, New York, NY, 1966, p. 165

35. McCrea, 'The Politics of Menopause', p. 118

36. https://www.standard.co.uk/lifestyle/london-life/international-womens-day-a-comprehensive-guide-to-the-feminist-waves-a3780436.html

37. https://news.psu.edu/story/141542/1998/05/01/research/natural-history-menopause

Chapter Two

1. Prior, Jerilynn C. MD, FRCPC, 'Clearing confusion about Peri-menopause' in *BCMJ*, vol. 47, No. 10, December 2005, pp. 538–42

2. Grant, M. D.; Marbella, A.; Wang, A.T.; et al. 'Menopausal Symptoms: Comparative Effectiveness of Therapies', Rockville (MD): Agency for Healthcare Research and Quality (US), Report No. 15-EHC005-EF, PMID: 25905155, 2015

3. Delaney, Janice; Lupton, Mary Jane and Toth, Emily. *The Curse: A Cultural History of Menstruation*, University of Illinois Press, Champaign, IL, 1976, updated 1988, p. 214

4. https://www.webmd.com/menopause/guide/guide-perimenopause#1
https://www.franciscanhealth.org/community/blog/first-signs-of-perimenopause
https://www.daisynetwork.org/about-poi/what-is-poi/

5. https://qz.com/1372767/twice-as-many-animals-go-through-menopause-as-scientists-previously-thought/#:~:text=Five%20animals%20experience%20menopause.

6. D'Souza, C. *The Hot Topic: A Life-Changing Look at the Change of Life*, Atria Books, New York, NY, 2016

7. Griffin, J. P. 'Changing life expectancy throughout history' in *Journal of the Royal Society of Medicine*, vol. 101/12, 2008, p. 577

8. Payne, Lynda. 'Health in England (16th–18th c.)' available from Children and Youth in History, Item #166, https://chnm.gmu.edu/cyh/items/show/166 (accessed 17 January 2021)

9. https://www.tudorsociety.com/childbirth-in-medieval-and-tudor-times-by-sarah-bryson/#

10. Mattern, S. *The Slow Moon Climbs: The Science, History, and Meaning of Menopause*, Princeton University Press, Princeton, NJ, 2019

11. Wratten, S.D., 'Reproductive strategy of winged and wingless morphs of the aphids Sitobion avenae and Metopolophium dirhodum', *Annals of Applied Biology*, Apr 1977, vol 85(3), pp. 319-31

12. https://www.goodnewsnetwork.org/grave-of-ancient-female-hunter-found-in-peru-andes/

13. From a conversation Alice had with Susan Bewley in July 2020

14. Shobeiri, F.; Nazari, M. 'Age at Menopause and its Main Predictors Among Iranian Women' in *International Journal of Fertility and Sterility*, vol. 8(3), 2014, pp. 267–72

15. https://www.mumsnet.com/campaigns/gps-and-menopause-survey

16. https://dianedanzebrink.com/menopause/

17. https://www.fourteenfish.com/

18. https://www.womens-health-concern.org/help-and-advice/factsheets/hrt-the-history/

19. https://www.nice.org.uk/guidance/ng23/ifp/chapter/Managing-your-symptoms

20.   Yokota, M.; Makita, K.; Hirasawa, A.; Iwata, T.; Aoki, D. 'Symptoms and effects of physical factors in Japanese middle-aged women' in *Menopause*, vol. 23/9, 2016, pp. 974–83

21.   https://medium.com/@adrianaveleznyc/menopause-its-longer-harder-and-hotter-for-people-of-color-d74f6293a53f
Gold, E. B. 'The timing of the age at which natural menopause occurs' in *Obstetrics and Gynecology Clinics of North America*, vol. 38/3, 2011, pp. 425–40
Avis, N. E.; Crawford, S. L.; Greendale, G.; et al. 'Duration of menopausal vasomotor symptoms over the menopause transition' in *JAMA Internal Medicine*, vol. 175/4, 2015, pp. 531–9

22.   https://warwick.ac.uk/newsandevents/pressreleases/hrt_prescriptions_lower
Hillman, S.; Shantikumar, S.; et al. 'Socioeconomic Status and HRT Prescribing: a study of practice-level data in England' in *British Journal of General Practice*, vol. 70/700, 2020, pp. 772–7

23.   https://www.menopausematters.co.uk/newsitem.php?recordID=198/Menopause-education-to-now-be-included-on-curriculum-in-secondary-schools

24.   https://thebms.org.uk/2018/10/bms-launches-new-find-a-menopause-specialist-service/#:~:text=The%20first%20set%20of%20applications,in%20the%20full%20press%20release
https://thebms.org.uk/find-a-menopause-specialist/
https://menopausesupport.co.uk/?page_id=60

25.   https://www.dailymail.co.uk/health/article-9614203/Half-doctors-arent-taught-MENOPAUSE.html

Chapter Three

1.   https://www.avonworldwide.com/dam/jcr:fcc532e4-f580-4c2e-9eb5-fa93b1290f2e/menopause-too-little-information-report.pdf

2.   https://www.bodylogicmd.com/for-women/menopause-symptoms/
https://www.ukmeds.co.uk/blog/what-are-the-34-symptoms-of-menopause
http://www.kwavi.com/wp-content/uploads/2017/05/Menopause_Symptoms.pdf

3.   https://www.acog.org/womens-health/faqs/having-a-baby-after-age-35-how-aging-affects-fertility-and-pregnancy#

4. Murkoff, Heidi. *What To Expect When You're Expecting*, 5th Edition, Workman Publishing, New York, NY, 2016

5. https://www.sciencedaily.com/releases/2014/04/140415203629.htm
https://pubmed.ncbi.nlm.nih.gov/21961722/
Harlow, S. D.; Paramsothy, P. 'Menstruation and the menopausal transition' in *Obstetrics and Gynecology Clinics of North America*, vol. 38/3, 2011, pp. 595–607
https://www.healthline.com/health/womens-health/why-is-my-period-brown#during-menopause
https://www.healthline.com/health/brown-vaginal-discharge#hormonal-imbalance

6. National Institute for Health and Care Excellence: https://www.nice.org.uk/

7. https://www.psychiatryadvisor.com/home/topics/anxiety/mood-changes-in-menopausal-women-a-focus-on-anxiety/
Bromberger, J. T.; Kravitz, H. M.; Chang. Y.; et al. 'Does risk for anxiety increase during the menopausal transition? Study of women's health across the nation' in *Menopause*, vol. 20/5, 2013, pp. 488–95

8. Born, L.; Koren, G.; Lin, E.; Steiner, M. 'A new, female-specific irritability rating scale' in *Journal of Psychiatry and Neuroscience*, vol. 33/4, 2008, pp. 344–54

9. https://www.menopause.org/for-women/sexual-health-menopause-online/causes-of-sexual-problems/hot-flashes
https://www.mayoclinic.org/diseases-conditions/hot-flashes/symptoms-causes/syc-20352790#

10. https://www.bhf.org.uk/informationsupport/heart-matters-magazine/medical/women/menopause-and-your-heart
https://www.medicalnewstoday.com/articles/317700#When-to-see-a-doctor

11. Weber, M. T.; Rubin, L. H.; Maki, P. M. 'Cognition in perimenopause: the effect of transition stage' in *Menopause*, vol. 20/5, 2013, pp. 511–7

12. Rekkas, P. V.; Wilson, A. A.; Lee, V. W. H.; et al. 'Greater Monoamine Oxidase A Binding in Perimenopausal Age as Measured with Carbon 11–Labeled Harmine Positron Emission Tomography' in *JAMA Psychiatry*, vol. 71/8, 2014, pp. 873–9
https://www.contemporaryobgyn.net/view/high-rates-depression-perimenopause-explained

13. https://nypost.com/2018/06/14/the-life-threatening-side-effect-of-menopause/

14. https://media.samaritans.org/documents/SamaritansSuicideStatsReport_2019_Full_report.pdf

15. Minkin, M. J. 'Menopause: Hormones, Lifestyle, and Optimizing Aging' in *Obstetrics and Gynecology Clinics of North America,* vol. 46(3), 2019, pp. 501–14

16. https://www.bjfm.co.uk/hormonal-headaches-in-pre-menopausal-women
https://www.migrainetrust.org/living-with-migraine/treatments/supplements-and-herbs/

17. https://www.menopause.org/for-women/menopause-faqs-hot-flashes
https://thebms.org.uk/2011/05/how-long-do-flushes-go-on/
https://www.menopause.org/for-women/sexual-health-menopause-online/causes-of-sexual-problems/hot-flashes
Bansal, R.; Aggarwal, N. 'Menopausal Hot Flashes: A Concise Review' in *Journal of Midlife Health*, vol. 10/1, 2019, pp. 6–13

Chapter Four, Part I

1. https://thebms.org.uk/2017/03/new-paper-professor-robert-d-langer-demonstrates-whi-study-errors-led-15-years-unnecessary-suffering-women/

2. https://www.readcube.com/articles/10.2147%2Fcia.s1663

3. Tata, J. R. 'One hundred years of hormones' in *EMBO Reports*, vol. 6/6, 2005, pp. 490–6
Stephens, Sahar M. and Moley, Kelle H. 'Follicular origins of modern reproductive endocrinology' in *AJP–Endocrinol Metab*, vol. 297/12, 2009, pp. 1235–6
https://jme.bioscientifica.com/view/journals/jme/55/3/T1.xml

4. https://www.urmc.rochester.edu/ob-gyn/ur-medicine-menopause-and-womens-health/menopause-blog/february-2016/the-history-of-estrogen.aspx

5. McCrea, F. 'The Politics of Menopause: The "Discovery" of a Deficiency Disease' in *Social Problems,* vol. 31/1, 1983, pp. 111–23
Casey, C. L.; Murray, C. A. 'HT update: spotlight on estradiol/norethindrone acetate combination therapy in *Clinical Interventions in Aging*, vol. 3/1, 2008, pp. 9–16

6. https://www.everydayhealth.com/womens-health/hormones/history-hormone-therapy/

7. Ritter, Stephen K. 'Premarin' in *Chemical & Engineering News*, vol. 83/25, 2005

8. Lewis, Jane. 'Feminism, the Menopause and Hormone Replacement Therapy', *Feminist Review*, no. 43, 1993, pp. 38–56. JSTOR, www.jstor.org/stable/1395068. Accessed 16 May 2021

9. 'Clinical Alert: NHLBI Stops Trial of Estrogen Plus Progestin Due to Increased Breast Cancer Risk, Lack of Overall Benefit' in *National Heart, Lung, and Blood Institute* (NHLBI), 9 July 2002

10. Mueck, A. O.; Seeger, H. 'Smoking, estradiol metabolism and hormone replacement therapy' in *Current Medicinal Chemistry – Cardiovascular & Hematological Agents*, vol. 3(1): pp. 45–54 https://pubmed.ncbi.nlm.nih.gov/15638743/#:~:text=Many%20 women%20receiving%20hormone%20replacement,to%20 smoke%20during%20the%20study

11. https://www.womens-health-concern.org/help-and-advice/ factsheets/hrt-know-benefits-risks/

12. https://www.nice.org.uk/guidance/ng23

13. https://mpoweredwomen.net/real-life/menopause-matters-me- saska-graville/

14. Schierbeck, Louise Lind; Rejnmark, Lars; Tofteng, Charlotte Landbo; Stilgren, Lis; Eiken, Pia; Mosekilde, Leif; et al. 'Effect of hormone replacement therapy on cardiovascular events in recently postmenopausal women: randomised trial' in *British Medical Journal*, vol. 345, 2012, e6409

15. Sifferlin, Alexandra. 'Hormone-Replacement Therapy: Could Estrogen Have Saved 50,000 Lives?' in *Time Magazine*, 20 July 2013 Sarrel, Philip M.; Njike, Valentine Y.; et al. 'The Mortality Toll of Estrogen Avoidance: An Analysis of Excess Deaths Among Hysterectomized Women Aged 50 to 59 Years' in *American Journal of Public Health*, vol. 103/9, 2013, pp. 1583–8

Chapter Four, Part II

1. There is an NHS factsheet about the types online. https://www. nhs.uk/conditions/hormone-replacement-therapy-hrt/types/ https://mpoweredwomen.net/medical/your-hrt-fact-sheet/

2. Stute P., Wildt L., Neulen J. 'The impact of micronized progesterone on breast cancer risk: a systematic review', *Climacteric* 21(2), 2018, pp.111–122

3. https://www.bhf.org.uk/informationsupport/heart-matters-magazine/medical/women/coronary-heart-disease-kills
4. https://thebms.org.uk/2011/08/hrt-is-good-for-bones/ https://www.nof.org/preventing-fractures/general-facts/what-women-need-to-know/#
5. Mosconi, Lisa. *The XX Brain*, Allen & Unwin, London, 2020, pp. 128–9
6. https://www.alzheimers.org.uk/about-dementia/risk-factors-and-prevention/hormones-and-dementia
7. https://www.daisynetwork.org/

Chapter Five

1. https://www.worldpranichealing.com/en/mantra/om-shanti-om/
2. Leon, Patricia; Chedraui, Peter; Hidalgo, Luis; Ortiz, Fernando. 'Perceptions and attitudes toward the menopause among middle-aged women from Guayaquil, Ecuador' in *Maturitas*, vol. 57/3, 2007, pp. 233–8
3. Mahadeen, A. I.; Halabi, J. O.; Callister, L. C. 'Menopause: a Qualitative Study of Jordanian Women's Perceptions' in *International Nursing Review*, vol. 55/4, 2008, pp. 427–33
4. Fitzpatrick, K. *Foraging and Menstruation in the Hadza of Tanzania* (Doctoral thesis, University of Cambridge), 2018
5. https://www.nytimes.com/1997/09/16/science/theorists-see-evolutionary-advantages-in-menopause.html
6. Minkin, M. J.; Reiter, S.; Maamari, R. 'Prevalence of postmenopausal symptoms in North America and Europe' in *Menopause*, vol. 22/11, 2015, pp. 1231–8
7. Jones, E. K.; Jurgenson, J. R.; Katzenellenbogen, J. M.; et al. 'Menopause and the influence of culture: another gap for Indigenous Australian women?' in *BMC Women's Health*, vol. 12/43, 2012
8. Hunter, Myra and Smith, Melanie. *Living Well Through the Menopause*, Robinson, London, 2021
9. https://triyoga.co.uk/blog/yoga/menopause-yoga
10. https://www.healthline.com/health/womens-health/benefits-of-a-girlsquad-and-female-friendships#Is-there-a-science-behind-female-friendships?
11. https://www.rcog.org.uk/en/news/cognitive-behavioural-therapy-and-mindfulness-can-help-manage-menopausal-symptoms/

van Driel, C. M.; Stuursma, A.; Schroevers, M. J.; Mourits, M. J.; de Bock, G. H. 'Mindfulness, cognitive behavioural and behaviour-based therapy for natural and treatment-induced menopausal symptoms: a systematic review and meta-analysis' in *BJOG: An International Journal of Obstetrics and Gynaecology*, vol. 126/3, 2019, pp. 330–9

12. Burch, Vidyamala and Irvin, Claire. *Mindfulness for Women*, Piatkus, London, 2016

13. *Journal of Affective Disorders*, https://www.journals.elsevier.com/journal-of-affective-disorders/

14. https://www.sciencealert.com/just-looking-at-photos-of-nature-could-be-enough-to-lower-your-work-stress-levels

Chapter Six

1. https://www.theguardian.com/society/2019/mar/26/long-sedentary-periods-are-bad-for-health-and-cost-nhs-700m-a-year

2. https://poets.org/poem/do-not-go-gentle-good-night

3. D'Souza, Christa. *The Hot Topic*, Short Books, London, 2016

4. https://www.health.harvard.edu/womens-health/why-does-alcohol-affect-women-differently
https://www.healthline.com/health/menopause/alcohol#5
https://megsmenopause.com/2018/07/02/alcohol-and-the-menopause/
https://www.endocrineweb.com/menopause-alcohol

5. https://www.mariongluckclinic.com/blog/causes-of-weight-gain-during-menopause-2.html

6. https://www.sleepfoundation.org/physical-health/sleep-and-overeating#

7. Herber-Gast, Gerrie-Cor M. and Mishra, Gita D. 'Fruit, Mediterranean-style, and high-fat and -sugar diets are associated with the risk of night sweats and hot flushes in midlife: results from a prospective cohort study' in *American Journal of Clinical Nutrition*, vol. 97/5, 2013, pp. 1092–9

8. https://www.heart.org/en/news/2020/03/23/soy-rich-foods-like-tofu-may-help-lower-heart-disease-risk

9. Wu, W. H.; Liu, L. Y.; Chung, C. J.; Jou, H. J.; Wang, T. A. 'Estrogenic effect of yam ingestion in healthy postmenopausal women' in *Journal of the American College of Nutrition*, vol. 24/4, 2005, pp. 235–43

10. https://www.nutrition.org.uk/nutritionscience/nutrients-food-and-ingredients/protein.html?start=2

11. https://www.webmd.com/digestive-disorders/news/20191028/could-more-coffee-bring-a-healthier-microbiome
https://www.ncbi.nlm.nih.gov/pmc/articles/PMC7105939/
https://www.gutmicrobiotaforhealth.com/whats-the-relationship-between-fermented-food-consumption-gut-microbiota-and-health/#:~:text=Compared%20to%20non%2Dconsumers%2C%20the,as%20protection%20against%20cardiovascular%20diseases

12. https://menopause.livebetterwith.com/blogs/stories-info/why-does-menopause-cause-leg-cramps-and-pains

13. https://www.nutrition.org.uk/nutritioninthenews/new-reports/983-newvitamind.html
https://www.nhs.uk/conditions/vitamins-and-minerals/vitamin-d/

14. https://www.nhs.uk/live-well/exercise/
https://inews.co.uk/news/health/walking-10000-steps-improve-bone-strength-283985
https://www.sheffield.ac.uk/NOGG/NOGG%20Guideline%202017%20July%202019%20Final%20Update%20290719.pdf

15. https://www.netdoctor.co.uk/healthy-living/a25407130/cbd-pain-relief/

Chapter Seven

1. https://www.nhsemployers.org/retention-and-staff-experience/health-and-wellbeing/taking-a-targeted-approach/taking-a-targeted-approach/menopause-in-the-workplace
https://www.dailymail.co.uk/news/article-6929515/There-4-9million-women-holding-job-age-50-rise-pension-age.html
https://menopauseintheworkplace.co.uk/menopause-at-work/menopause-and-work-its-important

2. Lewis, Rebecca and Newson, Louise. 'Menopause at Work: a survey to look at the impact of menopausal and perimenopausal symptoms upon women in the workplace', Newson Health Menopause and Wellbeing Centre, 2019

3. https://www.gov.uk/government/publications/menopause-transition-effects-on-womens-economic-participation

4. https://execpipeline.com/wp-content/uploads/2020/12/The-Pipeline-Women-Count-2020-1.pdf

5. Ibid
6. https://menopauseintheworkplace.co.uk/the-benefits
7. https://www.ipsos.com/ipsos-mori/en-uk/world-menopause-day-2020
8. https://www.cipd.co.uk/Images/menopause-guide_tcm18-55426.pdf
9. https://www.gov.uk/government/publications/menopause-transition-effects-on-womens-economic-participation
10. https://hansard.parliament.uk/search?startDate=1800-01-01&endDate=2020-09-29&searchTerm=menopause%20&partial=False
    https://www.rachelmaclean.uk/2019/07/04/rachel-reacts-to-momentous-decision-to-include-menopause-education-on-school-curriculum/
11. https://www.news-medical.net/news/20200602/Study-High-estrogen-levels-may-influence-alcohol-use-disorder.aspx
12. https://www.equalityhumanrights.com/en/advice-and-guidance/your-rights-under-equality-act-2010
    https://www.legislation.gov.uk/ukpga/1974/37/contents
    https://www.som.org.uk/sites/som.org.uk/files/Guidance-on-menopause-and-the-workplace.pdf
    https://www.fom.ac.uk/health-at-work-2/information-for-employers/dealing-with-health-problems-in-the-workplace/advice-on-the-menopause
13. See note 7.

Chapter Eight

1. Jackson, K. L.; Janssen, I.; Appelhans, B. M.; et al. 'Body image satisfaction and depression in midlife women: The Study of Women's Health Across the Nation' (SWAN) in *Archives of Women's Mental Health*, vol. 17/3, 2014, pp. 177–87
2. Gagne, D. A.; Von Holle, A.; Brownley, K. A.; Runfola, C. D.; Hofmeier, S.; Branch, K. E.; Bulik, C. M. 'Eating disorder symptoms and weight and shape concerns in a large web-based convenience sample of women ages 50 and above: results of the Gender and Body Image (GABI) study' in *International Journal of Eating Disorders*, vol. 45/7, 2012, pp. 832–44
3. https://www.beateatingdisorders.org.uk

4. https://www.vichy.co.uk/menopause-and-collagen-loss
5. Levine, Morgan E.; Lu, Ake T.; Chen, Brian H.; Hernandez, Dena G.; et al. 'Menopause Accelerates Biological Aging' in *Proceedings of the National Academy of Sciences*, vol. 113/33, 2016, pp. 9327–32
6. Mahto, Anjali. *The Skincare Bible*, Penguin Life, London, 2018
7. https://www.newfaceny.com/blog/how-does-our-nose-shape-change-with-age/
8. https://megsmenopause.com/2019/11/22/hormonal-acne-and-the-menopause/
9. https://www.jeffmorrisondds.com/blog-archive-1/2017/03/how-menopause-affects-your-oral-health.html
    https://www.avogel.co.uk/health/menopause/videos/mouth-problems-during-menopause/
    https://www.healthline.com/nutrition/menopause-diet
    Passos-Soares, J. S.; Vianna, M. I. P.; Gomes-Filho, I. S.; et al. 'Association between osteoporosis treatment and severe periodontitis in postmenopausal women' in *Menopause*, vol. 24/7, 2017, pp. 789–95
10. https://pantene.com/en-us/pantene-power-to-transform
11. Famenini, S.; Slaught, C.; Duan, L.; Goh, C. 'Demographics of women with female pattern hair loss and the effectiveness of spironolactone therapy' in *Journal of the American Academy of Dermatology*, vol. 73/4, 2015, pp. 705–70

Chapter Nine

1. https://www.thetimes.co.uk/article/the-gender-sleep-gap-our-new-survey-reveals-why-women-cant-sleep-jqk3729lv
2. https://www.nhs.uk/live-well/sleep-and-tiredness/why-lack-of-sleep-is-bad-for-your-health/
    https://www.rand.org/randeurope/research/projects/the-value-of-the-sleep-economy
3. https://www.hormone.org/your-health-and-hormones/sleep-and-circadian-rhythm
    https://www.psychologytoday.com/gb/blog/sleep-newzzz/201901/3-amazing-benefits-gaba
4. https://www.positivepause.co.uk/all-blogs/restless-legs-syndrome-is-it-ruining-your-menopause-sleep
5. Jones, H. J.; Huang, A. J.; Subak, L. L.; Brown, J. S.; Lee, K. A.

'Bladder Symptoms in the Early Menopausal Transition' in *Journal of Women's Health*, vol. 25/5, 2016, pp. 457–63

6. http://sleepeducation.org/essentials-in-sleep/snoring/overview-and-facts

7. https://www.independent.co.uk/life-style/gadgets-and-tech/news/netflix-downloads-sleep-biggest-competition-video-streaming-ceo-reed-hastings-amazon-prime-sky-go-now-tv-a7690561.html

8. https://thesleepdoctor.com/2018/01/05/menopause-affects-sleep/amp/

9. https://www.sleepfoundation.org/women-sleep/menopause-and-sleep

10. https://www.healthline.com/health/anxiety/calming-effects-of-passionflower#calming

    Yuan, C. S.; Mehendale, S.; Xiao, Y.; Aung, H. H.; Xie, J. T.; Ang-Lee, M. K. 'The gamma-aminobutyric acidergic effects of valerian and valerenic acid on rat brainstem neuronal activity' in *Anesthesia & Analgesia*, vol. 98/2, 2004, pp. 353–8

    Butterweck, V.; Brattstroem, A.; Grundmann, O.; Koetter, U. 'Hypothermic effects of hops are antagonized with the competitive melatonin receptor antagonist luzindole in mice' in *Journal of Pharmacy and Pharmacology*, vol. 59/4, 2007, pp. 549–52.

    https://www.healthline.com/health/magnesium-for-leg-cramps
    https://betteryou.com/health-hub/taking-magnesium-supplements-can-help-poor-sleep/
    https://www.getthegloss.com/article/why-you-need-magnesium-in-midlife-more-than-ever

    Rondanelli, M.; Opizzi, A.; Monteferrario, F.; Antoniello, N.; Manni, R.; Klersy, C. 'The effect of melatonin, magnesium, and zinc on primary insomnia in long-term care facility residents in Italy: a double-blind, placebo-controlled clinical trial' in *Journal of the American Geriatric Society*, vol. 59/1, 2011, pp. 82–90

Chapter Ten

1. https://helloclue.com/articles/cycle-a-z/vaginas-101

2. https://www.londonwomenscentre.co.uk/conditions/vaginal-atrophy#rt
    https://www.yesyesyes.org/vaginal-dryness/

3. http://www.repository.uhblibrary.co.uk/406/1/
Postmenopausal%20vaginal%20atrophy.pdf

4. https://www.nhs.uk/conditions/cystitis/treatment/
https://www.healthline.com/health/peeing-after-sex

5. Lewis, Jane. *Me and My Menopausal Vagina*, PAL Books, UK, 2018

6. See note 3

7. Crann, S. E.; Cunningham, S.; Albert, A.; Money, D. M.; O'Doherty,
K. C. 'Vaginal health and hygiene practices and product use in
Canada: a national cross-sectional survey' in *BMC Women's
Health*, vol. 18/1, 2018, p. 52

8. https://www.sleep.org/does-sex-affect-sleep/

9. Frostrup, Mariella (ed.). *Desire*, Head of Zeus, London, 2016

10. https://metro.co.uk/2019/07/13/keep-toxic-pressure-lose-weight-
away-masturbation-10253324/
https://health.usnews.com/health-news/blogs/
eat-run/2015/05/05/masturbation-as-medicine
https://www.elephantjournal.com/2016/11/the-masturbation-diet-
a-pleasurable-approach-to-curb-cravings-emotional-eating/
https://www.womansday.com/relationships/sex-tips/advice/
a1922/8-sexy-ways-to-burn-calories-110923/

11. https://thebms.org.uk/publications/tools-for-clinicians/
testosterone-replacement-in-menopause/

12. https://www.nice.org.uk/guidance/ng23/chapter/recommendations
https://www.bumc.bu.edu/sexualmedicine/publications/
testosterone-insufficiency-in-women-fact-or-fiction/#
https://thebms.org.uk/publications/tools-for-clinicians/
testosterone-replacement-in-menopause/

13. Barthalow Koch, Patricia; Kernoff Mansfield, Phyllis; Thurau,
Debra; Carey, Molly. 'Feeling frumpy: The relationships between
body image and sexual response changes in midlife women' in
Journal of Sex Research, vol. 42/3, 2005, pp. 215–23

14. Horvath, Zsolt; Hodt Smith, Betina; Sal, Dorottya; Hevesi,
Krisztina; Rowland, David L. 'Body Image, Orgasmic Response,
and Sexual Relationship Satisfaction: Understanding
Relationships and Establishing Typologies Based on Body Image
Satisfaction' in *Sexual Medicine*, vol. 8/4, 2020, pp. 740–51

15. Moran, Caitlin. *More Than a Woman*, Ebury Press, London,
2020

16. Forbes, M. K.; Eaton, N. R.; Krueger, R. F. 'Sexual Quality of Life
and Aging: A Prospective Study of a Nationally Representative

Sample' in *Journal of Sexual Research*, vol. 54/2, 2017,
pp. 137–48

17. https://www.onbuy.com/gb/blog/revealed-over-60s-sex-habits-in-2020~a245/

Chapter Eleven

1. https://www.dailymail.co.uk/news/article-8374181/Millions-men-suffering-partners-menopause.html
https://www.avonworldwide.com/beauty-innovation/innovation-centre/future-of-beauty/menopause-too-little-information-report

2. Rosenfeld, Michael J. 'Who Wants the Breakup? Gender and Breakup in Heterosexual Couples', in Alwin, Duane F.; Felmlee, Diane; and Kreager, Derek (eds.). *Social Networks and the Life Course: Integrating the Development of Human Lives and Social Relational Networks*, Springer, Berlin/Heidelberg, 2017, pp. 221–43

3. https://www.ons.gov.uk/peoplepopulationandcommunity/birthsdeathsandmarriages/divorce/bulletins/divorcesinenglandandwales/2019#number-of-divorces-and-rates

4. https://www.ons.gov.uk/peoplepopulationandcommunity/birthsdeathsandmarriages/divorce/bulletins/divorcesinenglandandwales/2018#

5. https://www.dailymail.co.uk/tvshowbiz/article-103226/The-age-gap-new-husband-If-dies-dies.html

6. https://www.ncbi.nlm.nih.gov/pmc/articles/PMC6257199/

7. Carey, Tanith and Rudkin, Dr Angharad. *What's My Teenager Thinking*, Dorling Kindersley, London, 2020

Chapter Twelve

1. Lupton, M. J.; Toth, E.; Delaney, J. *The Curse: A Cultural History of Menstruation*, University of Illinois Press, Champaign, IL, 1976, updated 1988

2. Foxcroft, L. *Hot Flushes, Cold Science: A History of the Modern Menopause*, Granta Publications, London, 2011

3. Lupton, et al. *The Curse*

4. https://www.theguardian.com/us-news/2020/aug/13/michelle-obama-menopause-account-spotify-podcast

5. Anderson, Gillian and Nadal, Jennifer. *We*, Atria Paperback, New York, 2018

6. https://www.vogue.com/article/gwyneth-paltrow-menopause-perimenopause-symptoms-hormones-mood-swings-sex-drive-goop-madame-ovary

7. https://www.resolutionfoundation.org/publications/happy-now-lessons-for-economic-policy-makers-from-a-focus-on-subjective-well-being/

8. http://content.time.com/time/magazine/article/0,9171,2019628,00.html

9. Campbell, K. E.; Dennerstein, L.; Tacey, M.; Szoeke, C. E. 'The trajectory of negative mood and depressive symptoms over two decades' in *Maturitas*, vol. 95, 2017, pp. 36–41

10. Brown, Lydia; Brown, Valerie; Judd, Fiona and Bryant, Christina. 'It's not as bad as you think: menopausal representations are more positive in postmenopausal women' in *Journal of Psychosomatic Obstetrics & Gynecology*, vol. 39/4, 2018, pp. 281–8

11. https://hbr.org/2019/06/research-women-score-higher-than-men-in-most-leadership-skills

12. https://www.girlboss.com/read/women-who-found-success-later-in-life

13. https://www.telegraph.co.uk/goodlife/living/over-50s-are-worth-billions-according-to-new-report/
https://www.hitachicapital.co.uk/media/1393/hitachi-capital-uk-silver-pound-report.pdf

14. https://www.premiumbeautynews.com/en/pro-ageing-let-me-be-me,13261
https://www.seppic.com/en/beauty-care-mag/pro-age-when-ageing-becomes-trendy
https://www.vogue.co.uk/beauty/article/menopausal-skincare

Epilogue

1. https://www.thetimes.co.uk/article/caitlin-moran-me-drugs-and-the-perimenopause-mpzn2cdh2

Bibliography

Abernethy, K., 2019. *Menopause: The One-Stop Guide: A Practical Guide to Understanding and Dealing with the Menopause.* London: Profile.

Arroll, Dr M.A. and Efiong, L., 2016. *The Menopause Maze: The Complete Guide to Conventional, Complementary and Self-Help Options.* London: Jessica Kingsley Publishers.

Burch, V. and Irvin, C., 2016. *Mindfulness for Women: Declutter Your Mind, Simplify Your Life, Find Time to 'Be'.* London: Little, Brown Book Group.

D'Souza, C., 2016. *The Hot Topic: A Life-Changing Look at the Change of Life.* New York: Atria Books.

Greer, G., 2018. *The Change: Women, Ageing and the Menopause.* London: Bloomsbury Publishing.

Henpicked and Garlick, D. (ed.), 2018. *Menopause: The Change for the Better.* London: Bloomsbury Publishing.

Kaye, Dr P., 2020. *The M Word: Everything You Need to Know About the Menopause.* Chichester: Summersdale Publishers Limited.

Lewis, J., 2018. *Me and My Menopausal Vagina: Living with Vaginal Atrophy.* London: PAL Books.

Lupton, M.J., Delaney, J. and Toth, E., 1988. *The Curse: A Cultural History of Menstruation.* Illinois: University of Illinois Press.

Mathews, M., 2020. *The New Hot: Taking on the Menopause with Attitude and Style.* London: Ebury Publishing.

Mattern, S., 2021. *The Slow Moon Climbs: The Science, History, and Meaning of Menopause*. Princeton: Princeton University Press.

McGregor, Dr A.J., 2020. *Sex Matters: How Male-Centric Medicine Endangers Women's Health and What We Can Do About It*. London: Quercus.

Mosconi, Dr L., 2020. *The XX Brain: The Groundbreaking Science Empowering Women to Prevent Dementia*. London: Atlantic Books.

Newson, Dr L., 2019. *Menopause: All You Need to Know in One Concise Manual*. Yeovil: Haynes Publishing UK.

Perez, C.C., 2019. *Invisible Women: Exposing Data Bias in a World Designed for Men*. London: Penguin Random House

Rogers, S., Sister, Dr D. and Hardy, L., 2014. *Your Hormone Doctor: Be Healthier, Happier, Sexier and Slimmer at Any Age*. London: Penguin Books Limited.

Reuben, D.R., 1969. *Everything You Always Wanted to Know about Sex, But Were Afraid to Ask*. London: W.H. Allen.

Showalter, E., 1987. *The Female Malady: Women, Madness, and English Culture, 1830-1980*. London: Hachette UK.

Sievert, L.L., 2006. *Menopause: A Biocultural Perspective*. New Brunswick: Rutgers University Press.

Tavris, C., PhD, Bluming, A., MD, 2018. *Oestrogen Matters: Why Taking Hormones in Menopause Can Improve Women's Well-Being and Lengthen Their Lives – Without Raising the Risk of Breast Cancer*. London: Little, Brown Book Group.

Tilt, E.J., 1868. *A Handbook of Uterine Therapeutics and of Diseases of Women*. London: Churchill.

Wilson, R.A., 1966. *Feminine Forever: A Revolutionary Breakthrough for Women*. London: W.H. Allen.

Resources

British Menopause Society: thebms.org.uk and their patient arm: womens-health-concern.org

Dr Louise Newson: menopausedoctor.co.uk

Henpicked: henpicked.net

Menopause in the Workplace: menopauseintheworkplace.co.uk

Menopause Support: menopausesupport.co.uk

Mpowered Women: mpoweredwomen.net

Pelvic floor health: gussetgrippers.co.uk

Premature Ovarian Insufficiency: daisynetwork.org

Sex toys: jodivine.com

The Menopause Charity: themenopausecharity.org

Vaginal atrophy: mymenopausalvagina.co.uk

Index

acne 55, 201, 204
adrenal gland 123, 154
Aetius 8
affluence bias 41
African-American women 40, 70, 300
African women 51–2
Afro-Caribbean communities 151
ageing 192–216, 298, 307
agnus castus 156
Albert the Great, Saint 9
alcohol 61, 62, 92, 142, 143, 145–7, 177, 194, 205
alcohol dehydrogenase 147
Alison 259
Allen, Edgar 83
Alzheimer's 101, 109, 296
Alzheimer's Society 109
Anderson, Gillian 288
androgenetic alopecia 208
anger 59–60
Annals, Claire 48–9
Annaradnam, Dr Amalia 96
antidepressants 49, 59, 61, 64, 65
anxiety 38, 49, 55, 57, 58–9, 95, 113, 123, 126, 136, 138, 142, 275
aphids 29–30, 32
Arab women 40, 124, 125, 242
Arif, Dr Nighat 39–40, 41, 44, 242, 267–8
Aristotle 7
Arroll, Dr Meg 29, 123, 267, 274–5, 277
Arthur, Karen 299–301
Asian women 150, 159
Association for the Cannabinoid Industry 161
atherosclerosis 107–8
Avon 267

Bach Rescue Night Remedy 231–2
Barber, Sarah 184

beauty industry 293–4, 298
Beauvoir, Simone de 17–18
Bellman, Gina 152
Bernard, Jessie 272
Bewley, Susan 33
Bigelow, Kathryn 291
bioidentical/body identical HRT 105–6
Biomedical and Environmental Sciences Journal 138
black cohosh 155
black women 300–1
blaming the menopause 68–9
bleeding: abnormal 58
    irregular on HRT 104–5
    post-menopausal 58
bloating 55
blood sugar levels 150
body fat 143, 149
body image 193–9, 251–2, 302, 305–6
body odour 55
body temperature 221
Bond, Jennie 296–7
bone density 66, 143, 161
    and HRT 85, 86, 88, 101, 107, 108–9
    impact of exercise on 157–8
Botox 193, 200–1, 302
Bowden-Smith, Andrew 270
Bradbury, Lynn 139
brain fog 55, 62–4, 95, 109, 156, 186, 251, 295
breast cancer 49, 58, 107, 119, 147, 156, 208
    HRT link 38–9, 83, 85–9, 92, 105
breasts 55, 65–6
breathing exercises 122, 129, 136–7
Brewis, Jo 172–3, 178, 179, 181
Brindle, Katie 308
British Heart Foundation 107, 108
British Journal of General Practice 41

British Medical Journal (BMJ) 93
British Menopause Society (BMS) 35–6,
    43, 44, 61, 70, 85, 87, 108, 251
bruising 55
Burch, Vidyamala 133–7
burning mouth syndrome 205, 206,
    214–15
Butenandt, Adolph 83

caffeine 61, 62, 147, 204
calcium 150, 154, 158, 206
Campbell, Katherine 290
Campina, Harriet 96–7, 214–15
cancer 58, 103, 143, 147
    breast cancer 58, 83, 105, 107, 119,
        147, 156, 208
    endometrial cancer 58, 85
Carey, Tanith 276
Caucasian women 159
CBD oil 161–2, 228
CBT (Cognitive Behavioural Therapy) 59,
    60, 126–9, 134, 139, 225–6, 228,
    230–1
Centre for Addiction and Mental Health
    at Campbell Family Mental Health
    Research Institute 64
Chance, Rebecca 262
childcare 32–3
childlessness 71–4, 227
children, effect of menopause on 274–6
Chinese women 40
CIPD 172
Claire 258
Clarke, Kate 282–3
clonidine 61
collagen 155, 199, 200, 203, 204, 205, 206
Collins, Joan 274
Collins, Laura 234
compounded bioidentical hormone
    replacement therapy (cBHRT) 106
concentration 62–4
conception 56
confidence 290, 293, 296–7, 302, 304, 311
Connor, Joyce 212–13
Constantine, Susannah 47–8, 216
contraception 58, 257
corpus luteum 26
cortisol 123, 138, 149, 222, 232, 235, 245
Coveney, Petra 131–2
Cunningham, Annie 42, 281–2

cures, nineteenth century 14–16
Currier, Andrew 16
Cusden, Tricia 211
cystitis 240

Daisy Network 110, 112
Damachi, Daphne 159
Danzebrink, Diane 36, 37, 44, 78–9
Darwin, Charles 31
dating 273–4
Day, Jody 71–4
death 12, 82, 93, 143
dementia 64, 109, 147, 186, 220
Dennis, Julie 173
depression 12, 55, 59, 64–5, 138, 155, 193,
    301
Derbyshire Fire and Rescue Service
    173–4
Deutsch, Helene 17
diet 58, 141–4, 148–52, 160
dieting 149–50
disability 42, 98
discharge 57, 242
disenfranchised grief 71–2
divorce 271–4
Dr Google 35
Doisy, Edward Adelbert 83
dopamine 64, 250
Down's syndrome 42
Doyle, Mary 98
D'Souza, Christa 29–30, 145
DXA scan 157, 159

Eames, Rose 97
Earle, Liz 44
early menopause 28, 40, 94–6, 309
eating disorders 195
eggs 26, 27, 57
Elvie 248–9
Emmenin 84
empathy, lack of male 102
employment tribunals 178
Enders Analysis 293
endocannabinoid system 161
endometrial cancer 58, 85
endorphins 157
Equality Act (2010) 178
ethnic minorities 39–40, 58
Evans, Sam 243–4, 246, 249, 252, 257
evening primrose oil 97, 156

hot flushes 54–5, 60–1, 62, 68, 70, 78, 97, 264
  alcohol and 147
  at work 167, 168, 171–2, 188
  CBT and 127, 128–9
  diet and supplements 155, 156
  HRT and 88
  and make-up 213–14
  sleep and 227
Howard, Sandra 94, 299
HRT (Hormone Replacement Therapy) 16, 41, 103, 303
  and Alzheimer's 109
  anxiety and 59
  benefits of 88, 99–119
  body identical 105–6
  and bone density 66, 85, 86, 88, 101, 103, 107, 108–9, 158
  and brain fog 64
  brave shame in taking 90–1
  breast cancer controversy 38–9, 83, 85–9, 92, 105
  breast changes 66
  commercial development of 84–5
  controversy surrounding 81–98
  during perimenopause 68
  and hair 13, 208
  heart disease and 85, 86, 87, 88, 93, 103, 107–8
  history of 18, 19, 83–5
  hot flushes and 61
  how long to take 106
  irritability and 60
  and migraines 68
  and night sweats 229
  and oral health 206
  and premature ovarian insufficiency (POI) 110, 112
  risks of taking 92–3
  and sleep 228, 229
  types of 103–5
  what it is 102–3
  see also oestrogen; progesterone; testosterone
Huffington, Ariana 291
Human Growth Hormone (HGH) 224
Hundle, Jog 177
Hunter, Myra 127–9, 139
Hyde, Jess 214
hydration 145

Hyposexual Sexual Desire Disorder (HSDD) 251
hypothalamus 60

ibuprofen 58
incontinence 55, 239, 246, 247–8
Industrial Revolution 11–12
Inge, Alexia 244–5, 294
insomnia 55, 57, 61–2, 142–3, 147, 217–34
Institute of Health Research, Canada 23
insulin 150
intelligence 295–6
International Journal of Eating Disorders 195
Ipsos Mori menopause poll 171, 180
iron 47, 51, 209
irritability 55, 59–60
itchy skin 49, 55
Ivens, Sarah 137–8

James, Jane Anne 115–16
Japanese women 40, 150
Jay, Dr May 37, 40, 41
Jewel, Dr Ateh 160
Johnson, Jilly 116–17
joint pain 55, 153, 155, 222–3
Journal of Affective Disorders 138

Kennedy, Annie 283
Kennedy, Paula 187
Kensit, Patsy 94–6
Kerr, Jim 94
Keyes, Marian 301–4
Kidman, Nicole 197
Kingsley, Anabel 207–8, 209
Kobson, Barbara 107
Koomson, Dorothy 45–7

LaFrance, Dr Marianne 207
Lane, Sheila 309
Langer, Robert D. 86–7, 88–9
learning disabilities 42–3
Leather, Professor Simon 30, 32
leeching, vaginal 15
legal rights 178
leptin 222
lesbian menopause 281–2
Lewis, Jane 240–2
LGBT Foundation 42

libido 13, 55, 115, 251, 252, 256, 257, 259–61, 268
life expectancy 30–1, 32
Lipman, Maureen 114–15
liver 146–7, 151
Logan, Gabby 304–6
London Hormone Clinic 96, 114
Look Fabulous Forever 211
Lowe, Pearl 74–6
lubrication 243, 244, 256
luteinising hormone (LH) 26

McCrea, Frances 19
MacGregor, Professor Anne 67–8
Mackesy, Serena 76–7
Maclean, Rachel 174–6
madness 12, 16, 287
magnesium 47, 152–3, 155, 229, 232
Magnus, Albertus 9
Mahon, Alex 185
Mahto, Anjali 199–200, 201, 202–4
make-up 210–14
#MakeMenopauseMatter 36, 43
Mansfield, Phyllis Kernoff 21, 252
Marinello, Giovanni 9–10
Marwood, Alex 76–7
masturbation 246–7, 252
Mathews, Meg 44
Mattern, Susan 31–2, 33
Matthews, Maria 232–3
Matthews, Sara 2
maturity 192–216, 254
Maudsley, Henry 13
'me-time' 128–9
Mead, Margaret 288
medical training 35–8
meditation 59, 60, 122, 132, 135–6, 137
medroxyprogesterone acetate 87
melanin 154, 200
melatonin 62, 228–9, 230, 231, 232
memory problems 62–4
men: effect of menopause on 265–74
    lack of male empathy 102
    male menopause 179, 257, 304
    sex 253, 256, 257, 258, 260, 261
    sleep and 224–6
menopause: average age of 28, 40
    definition of 11, 21, 26–8
    finding information on 34–5
    global experiences of 39, 123–6

mystery of 29–31
oldest recorded 28
road map of 25–44
symptoms 10, 14, 39–40, 54–80
through history 6–22
Menopause & HRT Discussion Group 115
The Menopause Charity 43, 44
Menopause Support UK 36, 37, 78
menstruation 7, 26, 27, 54, 55, 57–8
mental health 177
Meriwether, Joanna 259–60
metabolism 149
microbiome 151
micronized progesterone 100, 105
Middle Ages 8–11
migraines 55, 66–8, 138
Miller, Elaine 247–8, 249
Million Women Study (MWS) 86
mindfulness 59, 60, 122, 132–5
Minkin, Dr Mary Jane 65, 66, 125
Mirena Intrauterine System (IUS) 58, 104–5, 187–8
Mirren, Helen 291
miscarriages 74–6
money 292–3
monoamine oxidase A (MAO-A) 64
mood and mood swings 12, 48, 49, 59, 64–5, 138, 207–8, 235, 264–7
Moran, Caitlin 254–5, 310
Morgan, Kevin 229, 231
Mosconi, Dr Lisa 109
mouth, burning sensation in 55
MPowered Women 44, 90, 91
Muir, Kate 44
Mumsnet 35
Murray, Jenni 83
muscle mass 143, 157

Nadal, Jennifer 288
National Osteoporosis Guideline Group (NOGG) 158
nature 137–8
nervous breakdowns 64
Netflix 228
Neugarten, Bernice 288
neuroplasticity 295
New York Post 65
Newson, Dr Louise 38, 43, 44
Newson Health Clinic 164

premenstrual dysphoric disorder 65
Princeton University 289–90
progesterone 26
   crystalline 84
   HRT 74, 103
   micronized progesterone 100, 105
   perimenopause 146–7
   progesterone sensitivity 104
   and sleep 221, 229
progestogen 103, 104–5
prolactin 245
prolapse, pelvic organ 247, 249–50
pronatalism 73, 74
protein 151, 152
puberty 26, 27, 276, 308

raging brain syndrome 122
Rajasthan 125
Rameses II 20
red clover 155
Reddy, Donna 112–13
Rees-Mogg, Jacob 176
regulated bioidentical hormone replace-
   ment therapy (rBHRT) 105–6
relationships 263–83
restless legs syndrome 153, 223, 229
retinoids 203
Reuben, David 6, 8
Roberts, Rayne 146–7, 149, 153–4
Romans 6
Rosenfeld, Professor Michael 271, 272
Royal College of GPs (RCGP) 38
Royal College of Obstetrics and
   Gynaecology (RCOG) 36, 132
Ruth 186
Rymer, Janice 89, 90, 92, 93, 102–3,
   106

Saga Investment Services 292
sage 155
St John's Wort 65, 156
Samaritans 65
Samuel, Julia 254
Schumer, Amy vii–viii
Scot, Reginald 10–11
Scott Thomas, Kristin 286
Scurr, Dr Martin 240
sedentary behaviour 143, 156, 159
seeding 96–7
self-belief 215–16

serotonin 64, 138, 231
sex 88, 125, 235–62, 268
sex education 43
sexual orientation 42
Showalter, Elaine 13
Sieff, Mercedes 129–30
skin 155, 194, 199–204, 293–4, 298
   dry skin 55
   itchy skin 49, 55
   skincare 202–4
   skincare for sex organs 237–8
sleep: how it works 232
   improving 161, 229–32
   insomnia 14, 39–40, 55, 57, 61–2,
      142–3, 147, 217–34
   memory and concentration problems
      64
   night sweats 40, 55, 61, 68, 76, 97, 123,
      147, 221–2, 229, 233–4
   restless legs syndrome 153
   and sex 245
   sleep hygiene 229–30
   and weight gain 149
Sleepful.me 231
Sleepstation.org.uk 231
Smith, Jane 114–15
Smith, Mark 268
Smith, Melanie 127, 139
Smith-Rosenburg, Carroll 14
smoking 61, 62, 87, 205
social infertility 72
social media 195
soy-based foods 150
Spence-Jones, Clive 249–50
spicy food 61
SQoL (sexual quality of life) 256
SSRI antidepressants 61, 156
Stanley, Dr Neil 221, 230–1, 232
Starling, Ernest 83
Stephens, James 270–1
Stevens, Althea 77
STIs 257
Stokoe, Elizabeth 78, 188
Stopes, Marie 288
stress 136, 149, 160, 209, 222, 226–8
stress hormones 123, 138, 235, 245,
   246
sugar 148, 150, 152, 160
suicide 64–5, 78–9
sunscreen 202, 203

supplements 152–6, 161–2, 231
SWAN study 57–8, 193
sweating, night 40, 55, 61, 68, 76, 97, 123,
    147, 221–2, 229, 233–4
swinging Sixties 18

taste buds 50
teenagers 264–5, 276–7
teeth 204–6
temper 59–60
testosterone 26
    and acne 201
    effect of on hair 13, 208, 212, 213
    effect of stress on 209
    HRT 74, 100, 103, 105, 250–1
    and memory and concentration 62,
        64
    sex and 250–1, 256, 259, 260–1
    and sleep 229
Thomas, Dylan 144
Thompson, Dr Sandra 123, 125
thyroid gland 45, 46, 55, 80
tibolone 105
TikTok 41
Tilbury, Charlotte 211
Tilt, Edward 13, 15
tinnitus 55
Toledano, Dr Jan 114
traditional Chinese medicine 308
trans men 42
transdermal HRT 100, 104
Trotula of Salerno 8, 16
Truelove, Jackie 119
Tulleken, Dr Chris Van 152
Turkish women 40
Tyler Smith, W. 12, 14–15
type 2 diabetes 101, 143, 150, 154, 160,
    220, 222

ugliness, nineteenth century views of
    13
underwear 255, 256, 259
The Undoing 197
Urdu 40, 41
urethra 239, 240
urination: frequent 223, 236, 247
    incontinence 55, 239, 246, 247–8
    urinary tract infections (UTIs) 236,
        239, 240, 241

vaginas 236, 237, 238–9
    care of 243–5
    discharge 57, 242
    dryness 55, 236
    leeching 15
    oestrogen 106–7, 238, 242
    pelvic organ prolapse 247, 249–50
    vaginal atrophy 239–42
valerian 231
vasomotor symptoms *see* hot flushes
vibrators 245, 246
Victorians 12
visceral fat 149
vitamins: vitamin A 202, 203–4
    B vitamins 154
    vitamin C 155, 202, 203
    vitamin D 47, 150, 152, 154, 158, 159,
        209
Vogue 294
vulvas 237, 238, 239, 241, 242, 243–5

walking 138, 142, 159, 160
weight gain 55, 58, 92, 148–9, 222, 246
whales 29, 30, 32
Whitaker, James 269–70
WHO (World Health Organisation) 67
Wilson, Robert A. 18–19, 85
witchcraft 10–11
Wokoma, Dr Tonye 26, 27, 40–1, 42, 57,
    250, 251
    premature ovarian insufficiency 110
    taking HRT 103, 106–8
    treating menopause symptoms 58, 59,
        60, 61, 62, 64, 65, 66
Woman Count 2020 169–70
womb cancer 103
Women's Health Initiative 82–3, 85–9,
    109
Women's Health Initiative Memory Study
    109
Wood, Josh 210
work 163–89, 292
wrinkles 192, 193, 194, 199, 200, 203, 215,
    297

Yale University 65, 93, 207
yams 151
Yeotown 129–30
yoga 121, 122, 129–32, 223

Acknowledgements

There are so many to thank . . .

We're very grateful for the calm patience, intelligence and expertise of Dr Tonye Wokoma, whose ability to find humour rather than horror in a 7 a.m. panic text has been much appreciated. It goes without saying that any errors are down to us!

All the experts, politicians and women who took time out from their incredibly busy lives to advise us and tell their stories. We are especially indebted to Janice Rymer and Haitham Hamoda.

The running crew, where the idea of the book was conceived and nurtured, and who lent their assistance at its birth: Orlagh Collins, Caroline Corr, Sam Fuery, Sam Taylor-Johnson, Hannah Walker and Vic Yerbury.

For reading and encouragement: Gina Bellman, Penny Smith, Amy Gadney, Maria Matthews, Leah Hardy, Antonia Hoyle, Jill Foster, Rachel Halliwell, Sadie Nicholas, Eimear O'Hagan, Helen Carroll and Claire Coleman.

Consultant gynaecologist Sara Matthews, for the springboard of my initial diagnosis and subsequent illumination, and Saska Graville and Dr Stephanie Goodwin, whose fabulous seminar hardened vague resolve into action.

Brilliant agents Natasha Fairweather and Polly Hill.

Jason McCue for his many unprintable title suggestions and the final, acceptable one.

Illustrator Alyana Cazalet for so brilliantly encapsulating our ideas and bringing a blast of irreverent humour to the proceedings.

The talented team at Bluebird, who have carried us through the process with a tsunami of encouragement and support. Thank you Carole Tonkinson, Katy Denny, Jodie Mullish and Jess Duffy.